CHAKRAS
AND THE
VAGUS
NERVE

About the Author

C. J. Llewelyn, MEd, LPC, is a licensed professional counselor and marriage and family therapist. Her passion is combining the psychological, physical, and spiritual to heal trauma and facilitate personal and spiritual growth in her clients. C. J. is a trained Internal Family Systems therapist and is certified in EMDR (eye movement desensitization reprocessing). She utilizes polyvagal theory, energy psychology, and a knowledge of the chakras and subtle energies in her work. She is also a Reiki Master in the lineage of Dr. Mikao Usui.

To Write to the Author

If you wish to contact the author or would like more information about this book, please write to the author in care of Llewellyn Worldwide Ltd. and we will forward your request. Both the author and the publisher appreciate hearing from you and learning of your enjoyment of this book and how it has helped you. Llewellyn Worldwide Ltd. cannot guarantee that every letter written to the author can be answered, but all will be forwarded. Please write to:

C. J. Llewelyn, MEd, LPC
℅ Llewellyn Worldwide
2143 Wooddale Drive
Woodbury, MN 55125–2989
Please enclose a self-addressed stamped envelope for reply,
or $1.00 to cover costs. If outside the U.S.A., enclose
an international postal reply coupon.

Many of Llewellyn's authors have websites with additional information and resources. For more information, please visit our website at http://www.llewellyn.com.

C. J. LLEWELYN, MEd, LPC

CHAKRAS
AND THE
VAGUS
NERVE

TAP INTO
THE HEALING
COMBINATION OF
SUBTLE ENERGY
& YOUR
NERVOUS SYSTEM

Llewellyn Publications
Woodbury, Minnesota

First Edition
Fourth Printing, 2024

Book design by Christine Ha
Cover design by Shannon McKuhen
Interior art
   Figure 1
      The brain, in right profile with the glossopharyngeal and vagus nerves and, to the right, a view of the base of the brain. Photolithograph from 1940 after a 1543 woodcut. Wellcome Collection. Public Domain Mark (page 3)
   Figures 2–7 by the Llewellyn Art Department (original concepts by author)

Library of Congress Cataloging-in-Publication Data
Names: Llewelyn, C. J., author.
Title: Chakras and the vagus nerve : tap into the healing combination of
   subtle energy & your nervous system / C. J. Llewelyn.
Description: First edition. | Woodbury, MN : Llewellyn Publications, a division of Llewellyn
   Worldwide Ltd., 2023. | Includes bibliographical references. | Summary: "This book reveals
   the psychological dimensions each of your chakras hold and why you may hurt physically
   after experiencing traumas."-- Provided by publisher.
Identifiers: LCCN 2022055549 (print) | LCCN 2022055550 (ebook) | ISBN
   9780738773810 | ISBN 9780738773896 (ebook)
Subjects: LCSH: Chakras--Psychological aspects. | Chakras--Health aspects.
   | Vagus nerve. | Healing--Psychological aspects.
Classification: LCC BF1442.C53 L54 2023 (print) | LCC BF1442.C53 (ebook)
   | DDC 294.5/43--dc23/eng/20230415
LC record available at https://lccn.loc.gov/2022055549
LC ebook record available at https://lccn.loc.gov/2022055550

Llewellyn Publications
A Division of Llewellyn Worldwide Ltd.
2143 Wooddale Drive
Woodbury, MN 55125-2989
www.llewellyn.com

Printed in the United States of America

To Davis. Always.

Disclaimer

The material in this book is not intended as a substitute for trained medical or psychological advice. Readers are advised to consult their personal healthcare professionals regarding treatment. The publisher and the author assume no liability for any injuries caused to the reader that may result from the reader's use of the content contained herein and recommend common sense when contemplating the practices described in the work.

CONTENTS

•————————•

List of Exercises   xi

Foreword   xv

Introduction   1

Part 1: A Soulful Way to Embrace Your Body

Chapter 1: The Etheric You   11

Chapter 2: Finding the Sacred in Your Biology   25

Chapter 3: The Connection Between the Vagus Nerve and Chakras   49

Part 2: Healing through the Chakras and the Vagus Nerve

Chapter 4: Body and the Root Chakra   69

Chapter 5: Emotions and the Sacral Chakra   93

Chapter 6: Mind and the Solar Plexus Chakra   115

Chapter 7: Compassion and the Heart Chakra   139

Chapter 8: Connection and the Throat Chakra   153

Chapter 9: Spirituality and the Third Eye Chakra   167

Chapter 10: Empathy and the Crown Chakra   185

Part 3: Deepening Your Work

Chapter 11: The Spirituality of Healing from Trauma   201

Chapter 12: Soothing and Engaging the Vagus Nerve and Chakras   217

Conclusion   227

Acknowledgments   229

Recommended Resources   231

Bibliography   237

EXERCISES

·————————·

Chapter 1

Creating Sacred Space for Yourself   19

Imagine Safety   22

Be the Light Bulb   22

Chapter 2

Identifying Freeze Modes   30

Identifying Fight or Flight Modes   32

Identifying Safety Modes   34

Getting to Know You   41

Mindful Walking   44

From the Inside Out   46

Chapter 3

Breathing in Self-Compassion   55

What If There Were No Words?   61

The Emotional Is the Physical   63

Chapter 4

Body Scan   70

Get Grounded   81

Your Precious Stronghold   82

What You Can and Can't Control   85

Mindful Awareness of Your Root Chakra   88

Thank Your Body   91

Chapter 5

Buddha Belly   97

The People around You   99

Defining Emotional Boundaries Using a Value Circle   108

Emotional Boundary Script   113

Chapter 6

How Many Thoughts?   120

Looking into the Mirror   123

Fleshing Out Feelings   126

The Johari Window   130

Solar Plexus Meditation   133

Reality Is Relative with Relatives   136

Chapter 7

Be Still, My Beating Heart   142

From Five Senses to "Knowing"   145

Heart Chakra Connection   150

Chapter 8

Om Chant   157

Tapping the Energy Through   162

Forgiveness Prayer   166

Chapter 9

Soft Gazing   170

Stretching the Eyes   172

Third Eye Connection   179

Grounding and Shielding   181

Intuitive Writing   184

Chapter 10

Ventral Vagal and Crown Chakra Connection   187

Violet Flame Visualization   191

Empathy Visualization   196

Empathy Reflection   197

Chapter 11

Four-Way Breathing   210

Time for Deeper Reflection   214

Chapter 12

Move Differently   218

Waking Up the Spine   222

Breathing from the Heart   224

FOREWORD

———•———

T he brilliant connection between the chakras and the vagus
nerve for healing and self-care of our psychological distress
described in these pages by C. J. Llewelyn is truly cutting edge.
This represents a new frontier in the current movement to integrate advances in science with ancient wisdom and enhances our
understanding of mind, body, and spiritual health. The knowledge
contained in these pages expands our understanding of how to
care for ourselves.

It was when I had an office adjacent to C. J.'s that I first became
aware of the excellence of her practice and the breadth of knowledge she brings to it. While those were busy days, we managed
to steal a few minutes here and there to discuss ideas and trends
related to our practice. As a registered nurse, Michael Newton Institute Life Between Lives Facilitator, and a Reiki Master, I was aware
of the vagus nerve, the subtle energy system of the body, and the
chakras. I was familiar with clearing energy blockages to promote
physical healing.

During our discussions, C. J. shared with me how she had
used this knowledge in her psychotherapy practice experience to
develop an innovative healing approach. I was fascinated with her
ideas about the relationship of the vagus nerve to the chakras and
how she used this knowledge in her practice to promote emotional
healing and self-care. I was particularly excited about how she was

empowering her clients to use this information to aid them in dealing with their emotional reactions in their daily lives.

The integration of the chakras and the subtle energy system of the body is integrated with the nervous system of the body while the fetus is still in the womb. The teachings of Dr. Michael Newton revealed that we are Souls who join with a human body to live a life on earth to progress spiritually.[1] The Soul joins the body of the fetus sometime during pregnancy, usually around the fourth to fifth month. During that time, as the brain fully forms, the Soul brings its mind into synchronization with the brain. The Soul is pure energy and traces the neural pathways of the brain and learns the brain wave patterns of the fetus to achieve integration.

I first learned about the vagus nerve in anatomy and physiology class in college as I prepared to become a nurse. My classmates and I struggled to memorize information about where it was within the body and how it functioned. At the time, it seemed like one of the more complicated things we had to learn about the nervous system and very far from the clinical practice we were eagerly awaiting.

We learned that the vagus nerve is the longest nerve in the human body, originating in the brain stem and extending all the way down into the abdomen. A list of its functions could fill more than a page in our notebooks. The vagus nerve is involved in nearly every physiological action in the human body. It is the body's unconscious control system that helps regulate our internal organs to create balance and optimize our health.[2]

The vagus nerve also coordinates our bodily responses to keep us safe and warns us of danger. It is a key neural pathway of the

---

1. Newton, *Journey of Souls*, 269–70.
2. Peate, *Anatomy and Physiology for Nursing and Healthcare Students at a Glance*, 22–23.

body that transports information between our brain and the rest of our internal organs. Without our awareness, the brain scans the environment for signs of danger and alerts and prepares us to fight or flee. In extreme situations, it will shut us down. On the flip side, the vagus nerve scans for cues of safety, which allows us to become calm and open to socially engage with others.[3]

Later, I became a Usui Reiki Master. Reiki works with life force energy, called ki, that enters, circulates, and leaves the body through spinning or rotating energy centers called chakras.[4] While according to ancient wisdom there are many chakras within the human body, there are seven major ones, starting at the base of the spine and moving all the way to the top of the head.[5]

According to Reiki teachings, the main chakras are associated with major nerve networks within the body, which connect via the vagus nerve to all our internal organs.[6] The interaction between the chakras and the vagus nerve can be used for physical healing. I use Reiki to calm anxiety, relieve mild to moderate pain, ease nausea, and enhance healing.

C. J. has expertly developed an approach that combines current therapeutic modalities used in trauma processing to integrate healing between the chakras and the vagus nerve. The management and processing of emotions happens via the interactions between the vagus nerve and the heart, brain, and gut. C. J. carefully describes these interactions and prescribes self-care interventions to counter intense mental and emotional states. She has provided a road map for psychological healing.

---

3. "Vagus Nerve," *Psychology Today*.
4. Quest, *Reiki for Life*.
5. Alcantara, *Chakra Healing*.
6. Pfender, *Reiki Healing for the Chakras*.

The vagus nerve is a powerful nerve bundle. Recent research has revealed some findings that hold great promise for advancement in the field of mental health. This is a burgeoning field of research. Stimulation of the vagus nerve has been studied for its potential effect on treatment-resistant depression and ailments such as epilepsy, diabetes, and post-traumatic stress syndrome.[7] We've learned that the vagus nerve initiates a relaxation response after stress. Our gut can use the vagus nerve to send signals to our brain about how we're feeling. Gut feelings are very real.[8]

C. J.'s work has opened a new pathway to emotional self-care and healing via the chakras and the vagus nerve. This is a pathway that can lead us to a new way of thinking about our bodies, our being, our emotions, and our interactions with the environment.

—**Ann J. Clark, PhD, RN**
Michael Newton Institute Life Between Lives Facilitator
Usui Reiki Master

7. Caron, "The Vast Potential of the Vagus Nerve," *New York Times*.
8. Feucht, "The Vagus Nerve."

INTRODUCTION

———•———

T his book is about the capacity to heal yourself by understanding the restorative powers of your vagus nerve and chakras. These two separate systems—one measured by scientific principles, the other experienced through esoteric practices—bridge perfectly with each other in our bodies. Both systems have the power to restore your physical, psychological, and spiritual well-being so well that it would seem impractical to bypass one for the other as we work toward wholeness. If you possess a central nervous system, have ever struggled with anxiety, depression, or emotional dysregulation, believe you have experienced traumatic encounters in childhood or adulthood, or suffer from the results of trauma in your body, this book is for you. In fact, this book is for anyone who wants to stop running from their suffering that presents in the body (all of us) and start gathering information on how to heal themselves.

Our vagus nerve helps us to navigate our environment. It can determine our emotional well-being by gauging physical and emotional safety. As you will learn, it sends signals upward to the brain and back down to the organs and other systems with information about how to proceed with people and situations.

Our chakras are energy centers in our body. They can be felt when we incorporate subtle practices, such as meditation, yoga, bodywork, visualizations, breath work, or shamanic experiences, that slow our awareness down enough to connect with our body.

They sense our personal state of being and manage our way in the world with the acuity and grace of sonar waves. The chakras are also felt in our body as we go about our day; we usually just don't slow down long enough to notice. The overlay of these two systems is unmistakable.

What this book will do is explain why your body experiences the felt sense of your emotions and sometimes shuts down when more difficult emotions, such as fear, anger, or sadness, appear. I will explain how your vagus nerve and chakras play a role in this. I will also explain how the vagus nerve aligns with the seven main chakras in your body, and I will break down what psychological aspects each of your chakras possess and how they correlate with the vagus nerve.

The vagus nerve is the long fibrous nerve that appears to meander through your body. Though don't let its rambling appearance fool you. The vagus nerve serves as the unlocked gate to your inner peace. If you understand spirituality as a connection to the Soul Self within you, and how this Soul Self is experiencing being human, your nervous system is the pathway to staying connected to your peace.

Each branch of the vagus nerve sends and receives information to assist your life journey. The vagus nerve is known as the tenth cranial nerve, which originates in your brain. The vagus nerve manages control of the heart, lungs, and digestive tract. This nerve has a left and right side (bilateral) but works as one system. With the help of the brain, the vagus nerve retains "data sets" from experiences and the meaning you put to them. It registers events, then pulls from that information when it feels it needs to keep the body safe in present situations.

If we do not mend old emotional wounds—or change the "data sets"—that have been stored in our system, then we're defined by our past and bound to employ old coping strategies that may not be appropriate to the current situation. We are reacting to our past. We're not present to what is actually happening. This might be the simplest description of what trauma is.

Each time you push old pains back, you stuff them deeper into your body. The hurt then resides in your vagus nerve, organs, muscles, fascia, and brain. The "data set" is reinforced. That energetic reminder that is stored in your tangible self then resonates outward through the etheric energies of your body. Etheric in this case are the chakras that are sending and receiving vibrations. Unhealed emotional pain manifests into physical pain that is referred to as affect. Your system is screaming to be heard.

I am a licensed psychotherapist with a master's in family therapy. I have a background in healing trauma and working with people in recovery. I have been trained in approaches that process stuck energies through the body to alleviate the intensities I'm referring to. The modalities I use most with clients are body centered. They include Eye Movement Desensitization and Reprocessing (EMDR), Internal Family Systems (IFS), mindfulness, somatic work, and energy psychology, also known as tapping.[9]

The approaches in this book are what I use to help lay the groundwork for processing my clients' traumatic events. In my professional world, we refer to this as "resourcing." Resourcing includes using self-soothing exercises, grounding tools, and other calming approaches that assist your vagus nerve to engage in ways that feel safe. The exercises in this book are some of the resources I use with clients.

---

9. Shapiro, *Getting Past Your Past*.
   Schwartz, *Internal Family Systems Therapy*.

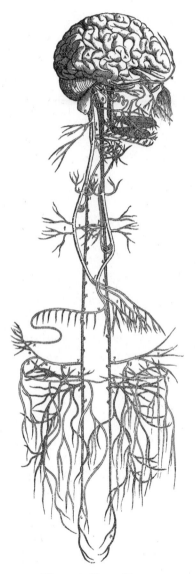

Figure 1: Vagus Nerve

Through the years—and because of my personal training with yoga and etheric energies—I have seen the overlay with emotional patterns and the chakras. I have developed skill sets around these energies to help my clients understand their bodies—both their chakras and their vagus nerve. I am also a Reiki Master trained in the Usui lineage by Dr. Ann Clark. This energy psychology reaches outward into my work depending on a client's comfort level. The yoga training in my young adult years helped me connect with the chakras in ways that were transformative for myself. Chakras are a wonderful entre into our psyche and physical well-being. They hold and transmit information if we listen. In short, I see the chakras as the light of our authentic Self that shines outward and works as sensors for our guidance.

I invite you to take this opportunity to become informed about your physiological makeup. When you understand your "wiring" you can identify the information it's sending and potentially calm it. If you are also able to understand your chakras, you can listen to your subtle energies for cues. Here, you can find the gateway to your Soul Self. When you know what is happening in your body, you know what is happening in your mind and spirit.

What to Expect from This Book

The biggest takeaway I would like for you to get from this book is to embrace the idea that your body holds over three-quarters of what you need to know about yourself in order to heal old wounds. Your brain is the filter that organizes and compartmentalizes that information. Your vagus nerve and chakras transmit that information.

In the coming chapters, I will break down the whats and whys of how your body and Soul Self are integrated through an explanation of your vagus nervous system and how it matches the etheric energies of your chakras. I will explain your vagus nerve through the polyvagal theory and how I've seen the chakra energy overlap. I will speak to both clinicians, who can see and maybe want to work deeper with these energies with clients, and readers, who want to learn more about their own healing and how important their body is in emotional/psychological healing.

What I can't do is define your inner energy for you, except to use the words *Soul* or *authentic Self* as ways to reference it. Soul Self is not a religious reference—unless that helps you. It is a simple word that describes a rather majestic energy we all possess. I can't reach in and get it for you and show you what you've been missing. It would seem that is part of the work we choose for ourselves when we get here. The work is yours to own.

This book is about helping you understand the tangible aspects of you as spiritual ones and the spiritual ones as tangible. It's about assisting in your psychological and spiritual growth by realizing the physical cues in your system. When you can find the pinnacle of the physical, psychological, and spiritual aspects of yourself, you can use the triad to help you through this journey your Soul Self wants to take.

In the first three chapters, I will talk about your vagus nerve and your chakras. I'll explain what the vagus nerve does and how an understanding of safety is paramount to you feeling a sense of connection to your Soul Self. Chapters 4 through 10 will break down each chakra. I will share how I see their psychological dimensions based on how they present in therapy sessions. I will also reveal how I see each of them aligning with the vagus nerve and how these pathways make sense for healing. You will be given self-soothing and grounding exercises. I will then conclude the book with basic information on what trauma is, how it is defined within my professional community, and provide resources for you to deepen the work with a professional.

The information about the vagus nerve I am sharing with you derives from my years of studying the polyvagal theory. The polyvagal theory was developed in 1993 by Dr. Stephen Porges.[10] Since then, his research has offered guidance to the therapeutic trauma community and has driven my own work. It is through the polyvagal theory that people are starting to understand why their physiological reactions appear to be emotional ones.

When I reference your Soul Self's journey on this earth, I refer regularly to the Newton Institute's qualitative research on life between lives.[11] This is also an overlay to my training as an internal family system's therapist. As a result, I will interchange the terms *authentic Self* and *Soul Self* on occasion, but both are referencing the inner light and wisdom within you.

While I offer insight and knowledge, I can neither define what your trauma is nor clear your trauma with this book. That would be irresponsible on my part as trauma healing takes time in safely contained environments with a trained and licensed trauma-informed clinician. With a licensed therapist, you can get an accurate assessment of your struggles, set healing goals, and develop coping strategies that will eventually help you alleviate trauma reactions that are stored in your body. The exercises in this book are resources for laying that groundwork.

Healing trauma or any past hurts is an "inside out" process, as you will learn. The memories stored in our vagus nerve present outward through the chakras. Energy healing can temporarily bring relief, but it does not eliminate how your body reads and

---

10. Porges, *The Polyvagal Theory.*
11. Newton, *Journey of Souls.*

copes with signals and meanings of lack of safety. Energy work can be done as an addendum to trauma therapy when it helps a person become more trusting of their body again.

When we grow psychologically, we stretch spiritually. Sometimes it's messy, sometimes it's uncomfortable, and sometimes it's downright painful. Yet, for every pathway you take, for every bridge you cross, it is a mile of adventure your Soul Self gets to experience. I hope this book informs and inspires you. At the very least, I hope it can provide a road map for your journey back to your inner light.

PART I
A SOULFUL WAY TO
EMBRACE YOUR BODY

———•———

CHAPTER 1
THE ETHERIC YOU

E verything about your physical self is here for a higher purpose, and this purpose is unique to you. Since your path is unique, so is your journey. According to the work of Michael Newton, PhD, Dr. Brian Weiss, and others, your authentic Self, or the Soul, chose the body that is currently reading this book.[12] Through decades of qualitative research, they have discovered that all aspects of your physical form are part of a greater plan. The inner light that shines within is imploring you to understand this. It's inviting your human self to connect to your authentic Self. Your authentic Self needs this physical body to complete its journey. When we can see things in this way, life takes on an exceptional meaning, doesn't it?

Your Soul is all knowing, all wise. It's pure essence. It understands things your psyche and body cannot. Like a wanderer in new lands, your Soul wants to experience this earth. It wants to be in relationships with others. It has plans for its own expansion and understanding. Ironically, this plan includes slowing down its frequency to fit in a tiny human body to do these great things.[13]

---

12. Newton, *Destiny of Souls*, 269–70.
    Weiss, *Many Lives, Many Masters*, 70.
13. Zukav, *The Seat of the Soul*, 137.

This body of yours also has an objective: to stay alive. Your physical form is of this earth plane. It seeks safety at all costs. You are just like any other animal on this planet. Before you can access the deeper realms of your being, which includes love and connection, your body must be guaranteed it will not be harmed. It's so good at its job that it has built-in systems to detect potential destruction.

When your body sees (or thinks it sees) scary things coming, alarm bells fire off. If the body has already experienced harm, it does what it's supposed to do brilliantly. It responds with even higher intensity than before, making sure you do whatever needs to be done to defend itself. Its preprogramming gets more and more refined at fighting, running, or freezing—all in service to the body's security.[14]

Humans are a walking contradiction. We are at once pure essence from a higher realm and gritty animal that strives to keep the species going. No wonder our human race gets so easily distracted and confused. The most important thing to remember is your body is not wrong. Its messaging centers might "get it wrong," but your body is a complex entity with the best of intentions. Acceptance of your physical self honors your spiritual one. Even when you're not getting what you think of as an optimal spiritual experience, you are always having one. Being on this planet and learning is spiritual.

So, how, then, do you manage to stay loving and curious about what is happening in your body to utilize what the Buddhists call beginner's mind when you get overcome with fear, pain, or self-loathing?[15] Beginner's mind is the capacity to see things as if for

---

14. Porges, "The Polyvagal Perspective," 116–43.
15. Suzuki, Zen Mind, Beginner's Mind.

the first time in a caring, attentive way. How do you find your peace when you have so much anxiety and too many negative thoughts? What do you do when you're depressed and struggle to get out of bed? Those very human experiences can be managed, which eventually allows you to thrive. I know because, as a therapist, I help people with this every day. With your intention to heal and the information that I can get you started with in this book, you can learn more about why your body reacts in certain ways.

When you accept that, at times, you need defense patterns to keep your body safe and can listen to them, you are honoring your built-in radar system. If you get overactivated in situations that don't require alarm bells, you can learn to healthfully calm yourself. If you don't get tense in alarming situations, because you are misreading cues, you can rewire your system for appropriate safety as well. This negotiation with the body then makes room to access a more peaceful experience. Your light will shine outward and more brilliantly than before.

Light Bulb Theory

I love to use the analogy with my clients that you are a light bulb. It's my own visual about what happens as you grow psychologically and heal. Simply stated, the brighter you burn, the higher "wattage" you draw into your life. You pull to you the situations and people that reflect your own brightness.

Brightening requires understanding what in your life no longer serves you. Those things may include behaviors or thoughts that keep you cycling in pain. Recognize—and be honest with yourself—about the patterns that keep you frozen in the shadows. Clearing old traumas in your system is at the core of this. It reveals blind spots and shines light into areas of your life you previously shut out.

Your luminosity shows itself in your chakras. They are the beacons of your Soul Self reflecting outward from your body. When you cannot access your Soul Self energy because of old fears, this affects the quality of light you give off. Your subtle energy is not easily measured and readily dismissed by science. However, it is strongly revealed through your presence. It is felt by you and others. Chakras, like a wattage in a bulb, are experienced.

These energetic centers are part of your complicated structure as a spiritual being in human form. When your body is physiologically activated by the meaning you put into a situation, the energy flows shift. How you manage your thoughts and ways of being in the world reflects through these wheels of light. This is most definitely not a mistake of nature, and these are definitely not two systems acting on their own. When we can understand that everything in the universe is interconnected, we can certainly see how our human and spiritual bodies are too.

Joan's Story: When the Physical Causes Emotional Distress

It's vital in the healing process that a therapist honor a client's own way of seeing the world. Joan's case is one of someone who had a direct experience with their vagus nerve that left them in need of connecting to their body but who would probably never feel comfortable with the concepts of the chakras.

Joan came into my office pale and uncertain. She had experienced a single event medical trauma and was suffering unbearable panic attacks. She felt absent from her body for hours after each episode and could not perform regular tasks because of this dissociation. The first day, she had to have her husband drive her to the session.

She appeared drained of her life force, like someone who had just come out of surgery or who was preparing to die. Her skin was gray. Clearly, she was scared. Her gaze would avert mine. She quietly sat down and glanced around, taking in the details of my office. I leaned forward and spoke, hoping my voice could register safety for her.

"Hello, Joan. Tell me how you're feeling."

"I've never been like this before," she said. "I can't sleep because I'm afraid I'm not gonna wake up. I spend my days sitting around because I don't trust what my body will do. I might fall. I feel hazy and sometimes," she glanced up at me, appearing worried about what I would think, "sometimes, I'm looking down at myself from the corner of the room. I don't want to see my friends. I feel like I've gone crazy."

"Okay," I said. "I can help you with that."

She held my gaze. "My pastor told me I shouldn't tell anyone about looking down at myself. He says people will think I've gone insane. He thinks I might have gone to hell and returned to be saved."

Joan told me she had a routine medical procedure under anesthesia that created an allergic reaction. For several minutes, she was dead on the operating table. She remembers talking to her father who had passed but doesn't recall details of the conversation. She does remember deciding to come back because she had young children to raise.

"The doctors say my—what do you call it—?" She glanced down at the notepad she was carrying. "My vagus nerve?"

I gave her a nod to let her know I fully understood what that was.

"It tripped or something," she said.

Smiling, I pointed to a three-foot-long poster of the vagus nerve on my wall. "That's what 'tripped' and probably shut down your heart."

"Hmm?" She stared at the lithograph.

"I call her Sheila," I said. That got a laugh. "I'm not a doctor, but I'm familiar with how the vagus nerve affects us. I think we need to get you acquainted with yours, so you can understand what's happening in your body."

Joan also told me her pastor feared for her soul. Since her father had been a bad alcoholic, the pastor believed the father was in hell, which is where Joan may have visited him. He told her she needed to repent. This terrified and confused Joan. She had been shamed by a person in authority whom she trusted. The work with Joan would require her to eventually trust her personal experience and find a narrative that was reassuring for her. But first, we had to get Joan to trust her body again since she was not able to function in daily life.

Clients who struggle with severe dissociation no longer trust or feel safe in the world. Their physical system misfires. This usually happens when they get distressed and feel threatened. Through various means, they disconnect from their body. This is usually a defense in early childhood that reinforces itself through the years, though anyone, no matter the severity of the trauma, can dissociate. As in any trauma work with a client, a therapist must assess for dissociative patterns and how severe they are.[16] It's also important to educate the client about what dissociation is and help them identify their patterns so they can safely ground themselves. In Joan's case, she had experienced a medical trauma that left her physically and emotionally confused. She needed to feel safe in my office and with me. I needed to provide resources for her to feel secure. To

---

16. Courtois and Ford, *Treating Complex Traumatic Stress Disorders*, 91–94.

start, I got her out walking during our sessions because she said she used to love to hike.

My plan was to get her connecting back to her body in the simplest, most familiar way any of us can—by putting one foot in front of the other and going. Walking is our built-in form of bilateral stimulation. Simply put, *bilateral* means utilizing one side and then the other of our central nervous system (and vagus nerve). It also resets our brain by engaging both right and left hemispheres and calms us. Walking involves the muscles in the lower abdomen, glutes, and legs, which gets all forms of energy effectively flowing. It also engages the lower chakras of survival, early attachment, and emotional connection.

I have an office on a small lake with a rustic path that circles around the water. Joan and I walked as she talked. Over several sessions, as we strolled down to the lake and around the circle, her voice became more animated. Her thoughts and speech grew clearer. One day, as she shared the memory of seeing her father, she froze and said, "I think I'm dissociating."

I asked her if she felt safe enough to look at me. She nodded. "Wanna try something?" I asked. "Let's do knee bends. Follow my lead?"

Giggling, she bent her knees when I did. After a few squats, I lifted my arms over my head, and she followed.

"Take in a deep belly breath, like I showed you, keeping the stomach muscles loose," I said, "and notice the scents around you."

Joan breathed in deep. "Honeysuckle. Grass," she paused for a second. "A little fried food from the restaurant down the road."

We laughed. "Now just move your feet and wiggle your toes. What does that feel like?"

She shifted the pebbles and dirt beneath her feet. "This is fun. You sure this is therapy?" She smiled and said, "I feel connected now."

"What are you hearing?"

Joan lifted her face to the sunshine and listened. "Some angry kestrels, a crow in the distance, a delivery truck." She then put her hand on her chest. "I also hear myself breathing."

Over the months of therapy with Joan, I had been gently helping her reengage with all aspects of her central nervous system by integrating everyday movements back into her life. Through walking, she was revisiting the natural sensation of working the left and right sides of her body. Through connecting with the smells around her, she was employing safety strategies of being present. "Belly breathing" helped her connect to her abdomen and midsection of her body, also linking with a sense of safety through feeling grounded. I was consciously engaging the parts of her vagus nervous system that employ safety.

I was helping her to ground through the root chakra, which is the energy of physical survival found at the base of the pelvis, through leg movement. "Belly breaths" were a connection to the sacral chakra energy of relationship to self and others. Hopefully this was also helping her trust and connect with me in safe ways. Breath opened her heart chakra, which was also reestablishing healthy heartbeats and engaging the safety aspects of the vagus nerve. As she spoke in ways that connected to her emotions, her heart chakra was opening and her voice was developing less depressed tones.

Joan had been told her near death experience was "evil" by those she loved or respected. She felt shame and confusion, which had intensified her medical trauma. While her personal experience of seeing her father was one of delight and love, she had been convinced by others she was wrong. It was not my job to tell her if her beliefs were right or wrong. It was my job to help her come to her own conclusions by reclaiming a strong relationship to herself.

We talked at length about her own interpretations of her experience versus what she had been told. Joan was getting good at reading her body's cues in relation to her thinking. Eventually, we did Eye Movement Desensitization and Reprocessing (EMDR) and targeted one of her strongest fears: the fear she had been to hell because she was bad. Through the processing, which incorporates bilateral stimulation, her natural belief system emerged. She was not bad, she said. She couldn't have gone to hell if she had felt so peaceful. What emerged was even more healing than she ever thought she would feel. Her conclusion was that her father was at peace and not in "hell," and she was not "crazy."

As Joan checked in with her body more often, she no longer experienced the intense punch she had felt in her solar plexus that engaged fight or flight patterns when she thought about "going to hell." She also seemed to rebound physically from the medical experience.

Never once were chakras mentioned to Joan. She does not employ such a belief system, and I would not have enforced that on her. However, Joan can now tune in to her body and trust what is being communicated as a way to ask for emotional guidance.

EXERCISE
Creating Sacred Space for Yourself

As we continue with this book, I would like for you to set up a place that provides a feeling of safety. There are so many ways to help yourself feel secure, and nothing is as primary as creating an environment that you can return to time and again.

Identify that place. This doesn't have to be anything elaborate or expensive. Sacred, in this case, is a place where you can go to honor yourself and have time alone. This place can be anything from an entire room to a corner of a bedroom to an area outdoors.

Sacred space has boundaries. It respects the physical, mental, emotional, and spiritual aspects of you. Sacred space allows you the opportunity to explore your innermost world undisturbed. It's your sanctuary where you can feel assured enough to get to know yourself better without interference. Interference doesn't have to be from other people. We can create all sorts of interferences. Busy time, laundry, distracting thoughts, playing with pets, social media, housecleaning, work, and texting are just a few of my personal favorites.

Do you already have a sacred space and didn't realize it? How can you make this place even more grounding for yourself? Here are some things to consider as you set up or improve your space:

- Incorporate colors or objects that are reassuring to you.
- Notice the emotions you feel around the colors you surround yourself with.
- Find a chair, yoga mat, or meditation pillows that you want and place them in this space.
- Alleviate distractions, such as phones or electronic devices.
- Be intentional. Understand how being in the space affects you.

I love plants and candles in my space; they calm me. Every time I write, I have a candle burning. I love the energy, so I make the intention to keep candles close by. Ask yourself what soothes you or inspires you visually.

In her book *Sacred Space*, Denise Linn provides suggestions and techniques to enrich your space. From clearing negative energies with the four elements to the use of color and light, she provides techniques from her own Indigenous background to help you establish your unique area.[17] I've recently revisited her work to create more sacred space in my own office as I started to write again.

Play around with what calms you. Be aware of noise. As much as you can, attempt to alleviate aspects that leave you agitated. Use favorite blankets. Honor yourself by holding your sacred space as you work through this book. Return to this space as you explore the exercises. This area will help you connect to the hallowed within you.

There is something else to consider. Your body is a sacred space. That sounds a bit contradicting if you've been working most of your life to disconnect from it but consider treating your body as the gateway to higher understanding, and do not beat it, starve it, stuff it, violate it, numb it, or shame it into submission. From this moment forward, befriend your body. Be lovingly curious with it. As you become more attuned through the reading of this book, you will be able to know your feeling state and identify your needs.

---

17. Linn, *Sacred Space*, 277.

EXERCISE
Writing Prompt: Imagine Safety

Another way to approach this book is to get a journal, pens, and some colored pencils. Find something you can have fun with, like a journal with no lines. In many ways, this journal will be your sacred space as well.

This particular journal prompt requires your colored pencils. It's intended for you to deepen the connection to that which feels secure around you. With that in mind, here goes your first writing exercise:

- Think of a safe, secure, or peaceful place you love to go. This can be in life or your imagination.
- Allow yourself to feel the emotions that come up as you see yourself in this sacred place. Notice the sensations in your body.
- As these feelings come up, take out the pencil colors that represent those feelings and just draw with them in whichever way feels good. Color represents feelings in this case, so use your imagination and find the colors that feel appropriate to your experience right now. Later on, return to this collection of color and notice what you feel and where you are feeling it.

EXERCISE
Writing Prompt: Be the Light Bulb

Moving up in "wattage" requires understanding what you would like to pull into your life that is safe and good. The first step in achieving change is to imagine something you would like to have. Even if you don't feel you have safety in your life right now, with work, it can be achieved. Using your journal, explore the following writing prompt.

- Who is safe for you in your life right now?
- How do you imagine a safer, calmer life would look like?
- Where do you feel the experience of safety in your body?

Summary

Safety is at the core of thriving as a human being. Safety is not just a physical experience; it is an emotional, psychological, and social one as well. You can even feel spiritually unsafe if your reality of what is spiritual is derided by another. While it is harder to understand when you are threatened on these more etheric levels, you can turn to your body to listen for cues of what feels right and what doesn't. Safety and lack thereof is felt there.

When you do not feel safe, it is hard to thrive in other aspects of your life. You spend most of your time in pursuit of safety, which makes it difficult to connect. Creating as much safety for yourself, even understanding the importance of safety, is key to thriving emotionally.

CHAPTER 2
FINDING THE SACRED
IN YOUR BIOLOGY

•———————————•

O ur vagus nerve is a long branch of neuronal fibers that extends the length of your torso. It connects many areas of your body, including the brain, neck, facial muscles, inner ear, heart, lungs, digestive system, and spine. It is part of your central nervous system.[18] Think of the vagus nerve as your personal navigation system. It's the steering wheel, brakes, accelerator, and electronic safety detections of your body.

This nerve is part of the autonomic nervous system, which keeps your heart beating and your lungs breathing without you paying attention. This is important to know later as you learn to identify and manage your breathing and heart rate and understand how these bodily responses are affecting your emotions and state of well-being.

With the help of the brain, the vagus nerve is constantly receiving and sending safety cues. Every mammal in the animal kingdom works things out utilizing this system. They possess the same physical construct you have. The difference is you have a triune, or three-tiered brain, that allows for higher reasoning. Your human brain

---

18. Netter, *Atlas of Human Anatomy*, 125.

helps you break down your conceptual, emotional, and physical experiences.[19]

Imagine your brain like a three-layered cake, one layer resting on top of the other. The lowest part of the brain is referred to as the "reptilian brain." It connects directly to the spinal cord. The reptilian brain is fully developed at birth. It's constantly working whether you're sleeping or awake. It controls instinctive behaviors and the autonomic responses of your body. The reptilian brain generates reflexes. It reacts swiftly to keep the body alive.

The middle tier of the brain is the "emotional brain." This part of the brain allows you to experience what you like, love, and feel connected to. The emotional brain holds your reward signals. Those signals play a role in pursuits of pleasure and pain. It also plays a big role in relationships. This part of the brain possesses the hippocampus, thalamus, and amygdala. The hippocampus stores long-term memory. The thalamus registers safety and danger. The amygdala sends signals of threat to the rest of the system.

On top rests the largest layer. This is the neocortex, or the "higher reasoning" brain. The higher reasoning brain is where elevated concepts are born. This part of your brain is spiritual, creative, empathetic, and "bigger picture."

If you are looking at the brain from the front, the brain has two sections: the left and right.[20] The right brain is the intuitive, bigger picture, and imaginal aspect. The left is linear and analytical. The right neocortex is fully developed at birth. This part of our brain holds onto memories in an implicit way. Implicit is sensing and feeling. The left part develops through childhood and into early adulthood. This part works through memory in chronological ways. This

---

19. Ogden and Fisher, *Sensorimotor Psychotherapy*, 185.
20. McGilchrist, *The Master and his Emissary*, 20.

is why some people say, "I don't have a memory of this, but it feels like something might have happened when I was really young," or "It just feels good to think of being with my grandparents, even though I don't have a memory of them."

Polyvagal Theory and Your Body

The vagus nerve and the brain are the wiring that attempts to keep you out of harm's way. As we have been discussing, if your body is not safe, it's impossible to feel calm, loving, or connected. Dr. Stephen Porges brought this to light when he developed the polyvagal theory.[21] What started as his research to help infants became fully embraced by trauma therapists.

Porges's work burgeoned in the mental health field because it provided answers to what trauma therapists were seeing—that the difficulty in self-soothing, perception of emotional safety, and reactive patterns was not a personality weakness.[22] Feeling terrified in the face of calm, experiencing shutdown during a scary experience, his theory explains, is a result of miscues in the central nervous system. Those miscues are founded in past experiences and how they are stored in your system. As his work was introduced throughout the medical community, trauma experts in the mental health field saw something important at play. Suddenly, there was a biological understanding of emotional behaviors.

It's important for you to have agency over your body and to embrace the messages it is sending so you can accurately engage in your life. In order to do this, you need to understand what is happening in your system. There is emotional liberation when you can recognize and trust what your physiological signals are telling

---

21. Porges, *The Polyvagal Theory*, 17.
22. Porges, "Orienting in a Defensive World," 301–318.

you. Identifying what is happening in your body allows you to be kinder to yourself and to speak to and treat yourself with understanding. So, let's break down your biology with the help of the polyvagal theory.

If you looked straight on at the vagus nerve, you would see two branches on the left and right side. This matches up with the two sides of the brain. Both sides of the brain and the vagus nerve work in tandem, or bilaterally, favoring various functions but combining strengths.

Looking at the vagus nerve from the side, as you can see in figure 1, you will see three different branches. These three branches play distinct roles in helping you navigate your world. These include the dorsal, sympathetic, and ventral vagus nerves. Let's break them down.

Dorsal Vagus: The Shutdown Nerve

The most ancient branch of the nervous system is the dorsal vagal nerve. It's roughly five hundred million years old.[23] Just like all creatures possess limbic (reptilian) brain functioning, your vagus has within it a dorsal vagal branch that performs basic functions for the body. The dorsal is a fin on the back of mammalian sea creatures like dolphins. Perhaps this will help you remember that the dorsal vagal nerve is on the back side of your own nervous system.

In times of overwhelming stress, the dorsal vagal will shut us down. It can do this through irregular and heavy sleep patterns, dissociating, or passing out. It will release your bowels or bladder, as it is attached to your digestive organs. Once, when I was working with a young man who had served in the armed forces, he

---

23. Porges, *The Polyvagal Theory*, 159.

told me he released his bowels in his pants during his first battle. When I explained that was a common response of his central nervous system—and described what his dorsal vagal nerve does—he smiled. His belief had been he was cowardly. The fact is his body registered a lack of safety (does it get more unsafe than being shot at?) and was attempting to shut him down.

I mentioned dissociation in the description of Joan's case in the previous chapter. When we dissociate, we are not fully in our bodies. In chapter 11, I will discuss more about dissociation, why dissociation happens, and how to identify your particular patterns. I will show you some techniques for calming and reorienting yourself. For now, know that on many levels we all experience some level of dissociation depending on the coping mechanisms that formed in our lives.[24]

When we have no ability to escape a dangerous situation—or what our guidance system perceives as dangerous—the dorsal vagal plays possum for us. It shuts us down. This helps our system conserve important energy when we have no recourse for safety. When you hear the term *fight, flight, or freeze*, this is what we know of as the "freeze" response.[25]

The part of the country I live in has been hit with tornadoes and floods lately. Many of my clients whose homes were damaged are reporting feeling disconnection and malaise. They want to lay around, sleep, and not see people. They don't meet the clinical criteria for depression; they just don't have the strength to engage much. They are at once overstimulated and exhausted. After reconstructing homes or finding new places to live or negotiating with insurance, they have crumpled into a state of exhaustion (dorsal vagal collapse). By helping them understand that this is a normal

---

24. Paulsen, *Looking Through the Eyes of Trauma and Dissociation*, 46.

25. Porges, *Polyvagal Safety*, 140.

response to being overwhelmed—that their vagus nerve is reading the body needs to conserve energy—they stop shaming themselves into action again and take some time to rest.

It's important for you to recognize when your body experiences this kind of shutdown so you can respond to it in supportive ways. Then you can give yourself what you need. When your body goes into a "freeze" mode, you cannot simply jump back out into calm ways of connecting with others as if you are already safe. It takes time for your system to move from a reading of danger to a reading of safety mode.[26] From a dorsal vagal response, your body works its way into the more active part of the vagus nerve: the sympathetic nervous system.

EXERCISE
Writing Prompt: Identifying Freeze Modes

Take a few minutes and write in your journal about the occasions you've experienced a dorsal vagal shutdown. Knowing what is happening is the first step to caring for and nurturing yourself.

Do you remember a time when your body collapsed and did not get up? What happened that caused you to collapse? What made you feel unsafe? Sometimes, we don't collapse but our body sends signals it's time to sleep when it's not, such as incessant yawning or drowsiness. What happened that caused the drowsiness? What made you feel unsafe?

What nurturing, safe ways did you work back to active engagement after a dissociative experience? These can look like imagining yourself moving before you actually move again or reaching for calming scents or soft materials to engage your senses.

---

26. Dana, *The Polyvagal Theory in Therapy*, 33.

Sympathetic Nerve: The Fight or Flight Nerve

The second branch of the vagus nerve is the sympathetic nervous system. It originates in the lumbar and thoracic areas of the spine. This branch of the system is roughly four hundred million years old. This nerve creates your "fight or flight" response when you're feeling unsafe.[27] It keeps you alert and signals when danger is nearby so you can run from or fight the threat.

When danger is perceived, the sympathetic part of the vagus nerve activates the hypothalamic-pituitary-adrenal (HPA) axis, which sends cortisol to your system. This process tightens the muscles to prepare for a threat. Heart rate increases because it is harder for the blood to access muscles when they are tight. The stimulation of the sympathetic nervous system keeps you alert to danger. This is a natural physiological response when there is a threat to your welfare.

However, this system can be put into overdrive by modern living and a stressful lifestyle. Rush hour traffic is the first example that comes to mind. Hurrying up to go slow puts the brakes and the accelerator on our system, doesn't it? Regular work deadlines, living in unsafe environments, or frequent negative self-talk are some examples of how you can keep the sympathetic nervous system "churning." Constant agitation of the fight or flight response has a deleterious effect since this system is meant to create short bursts and not long-term tension.

When we are raised in a violent environment, the sympathetic nervous system is constantly aroused because it has been conditioned to be on high alert.[28] To keep secure, we are watching and

---

27. Porges, "The Polyvagal Theory," 160.

28. Ogden and Fisher, *Sensorimotor Psychotherapy*, 225.

deciphering the moods of caretakers. It's not just a lack of bodily safety that causes stress. Emotional inconsistency creates fear too. If the family environment is chaotic, verbally or physically abusive, or neglectful, then the children are in endless disarray. Daily they gauge the mercurial moods of the adults or try to decipher inconsistent words that don't align with behaviors. When a child's system is in a regular state of fight or flight, over time the cortisol depletes from the adrenal glands and adult fatigue issues set in years later.[29]

Understanding how your regular behaviors, thoughts, schedules, and self-care contribute to the health of your central nervous system is core to your overall health. When you can determine that you're feeling anxious or fearful, you can calm yourself by working your system into feeling safe again.

EXERCISE
Writing Prompt: Identifying Fight or Flight Modes

As you get to know your body through tuning into your vagus nerve, it's important to understand how it was asked to perform in childhood. This journaling exercise is intended to have you reflect on this. If these questions become too upsetting or intense, please feel free to skip them.

- Did your family represent any of the previously mentioned descriptors of lack of safety?
- What made you feel unsafe growing up?
- Have you experienced unexplained fatigue in your life?
- Do you remember a time when you felt the fight or flight response? In what ways did you work into a sense of safety afterward?

---

29. Wilson, *Adrenal Fatigue*, 48.

Ventral Vagal Nerve:
The Social Engagement "Safety" Nerve

The third branch of the vagus nerve is the ventral vagus nerve. It is developmentally the "youngest" of the three branches at two hundred million years old. This section is located in the front of your body and regulates your ability to engage with people. It is the "face to heart" connection. For humans to feel secure, a relationship to others is vital. All mammals have a vagus nerve. It is what differentiates us from reptiles, which do not need to band together to survive.[30]

The ventral vagal nerve attaches to your heart and is an important driver of frequency and time between beats. It also connects to and affects your respiratory system, which controls your breathing patterns. Heart beats and breaths are interrelated when it comes to feeling stimulated or calm, which impacts mood.

Facial expressions are a strong indicator to others if you are approachable. The ventral vagal nerve runs deep into your jaw, mouth, cheeks, eyes, and forehead muscles and helps you send signals to others through expression and sounds. Smiles or laughter clearly indicate you're open to connect. Furrowed brows, downward turned lips, or a lowered head says you're not available.

Your eyes are also controlled by this nerve. Cast upward and meeting another's gaze indicates a willingness to communicate. Cast downward or looking away says you are disconnecting. This provides social cues to engage or withdraw. We are all more apt to approach someone who is cheerful and looking at us than someone who is frowning, gritting their teeth, and looking away.

---

30. Porges, *The Polyvagal Theory*, 133.

The ventral vagal nerve also connects to your middle ear. This helps you make sense of another's tone of voice, called prosody. High-pitched voices usually mean someone is in danger. Low-pitched voices may indicate anger. Midranges of voice are more associated with safety. Think of a time you heard someone raise their voice. What did you feel? What about a time someone smiled at you and greeted you in a calm matter? Consistency of voice and facial expression helps us gauge our acceptance by people. Have you ever experienced mixed messages from a person whose voice and expressions didn't match up? If someone speaks in a flat, low voice but is smiling, we decipher this as confusing. Are they safe or not? They "look" happy but don't "sound" happy.

EXERCISE
Writing Prompt: Identifying Safety Modes

This journal prompt is designed to help increase awareness of the emotional messages through your system. Check in with your body before you begin to write. Pull in some deep breaths and give yourself a moment before you begin.

- Are there areas in your body that feel calm? Where are they?
- What are you noticing about that calmness? Relaxed muscles? Soft breathing?
- Are you aware of any places in your body that feel tense or tight? If so, look around your sacred space and remind yourself that you are safe. How do you feel when you do this?
- Who are the people in your life you feel calm and safe around? What do you notice about your body when you are with them?

- Who do you not feel safe with? What do you notice about your body when you are with those people?

Driving the Vagus Nerve

While it sounds like being engaged with the ventral vagus is all good and the dorsal vagal is all bad, that is not the case. Your system regulates by utilizing more than one branch depending on what is happening in your environment or even the meaning you apply to a situation. An example might be the emergency room doctor who needs to stay calm and communicative while operating on a triage patient. They are using both their ventral vagal activity of being present and their sympathetic branch because they are on heightened alert. Another example of more than one branch engaging would be during sex when we feel safe with our partner. We experience both dorsal vagal and ventral vagal engagement.

Your "wiring" is always serving your safety needs. Keeping attuned helps you effectively negotiate what is currently happening in your life. This ability to be present plays the biggest role in your own resiliency. Like the self-driving safety features in a car, the system adjusts then readjusts. There are techniques to employ to help your system maneuver. As mentioned, it can take time and effort to bring yourself from a state of high alert (sympathetic) to safety (ventral), or a state of shutdown (dorsal) to safety (ventral). Breathing deeply is just one of those ways we naturally modulate ourselves. Talking to a safe friend with a caring voice may be another. Being able to identify safety markers and knowing what they are is helpful. The following are some examples of what safety markers are and how to use them.

Body Markers

The first marker for safety involves examining how your body is feeling and responding to your surroundings. Approach this process with kindness and acceptance.

Check your breathing. How are you pulling breaths into your body? Where do the breaths fall in your lungs? How steady do the breaths feel?

Observe your muscles. What do the muscles in your neck and jaw feel like? Are they tight or soft? Are you clenching your jaw? Notice the muscles that run along your spine and down to your hips. How do the muscles in your abdomen feel?

What are your limbs doing? Are your shoulders and arms relaxed or tense? What is the posture in your torso and shoulders? What are your legs doing? Are they crossed or shaking? Check your fingers and palms. How do they feel?

As you become more connected to the markers of your body, notice the presence of your placement in your seat. Be aware of the sensations of your back and legs in your chair. When you are driving, notice how you hold the steering wheel. When you walk, is your head down? Are you observing your surroundings or walking rapidly without looking up?

Emotional Markers

The second marker for safety is to observe how you are feeling emotionally. This is not so much a mental process (as many people believe) but a physical one. The markers of your body are very much interwoven into the emotional markers.

Are you worried? Sad? Confused? Are you experiencing happiness? Joy? Where do you feel these emotions in your body? If you're experiencing difficult emotions, breathe into the part of your body where you're feeling them.

Continue to notice the feeling states as you simultaneously check body and emotions. Look curiously at the combination of physical and emotional.

Even if you are struggling to connect emotion with the body, stay curious. Observe. Notice thoughts that are being applied as you go through this exercise. Stay curious and thank your body for this deeper information.

Environmental Markers

The third marker is to explore your environment. Check for facts that confirm safety.

Look around you. Where are you and who are you with? Are you with kind and supportive people? Do you feel engaged with these people or disengaged?

Are you in a safe environment? Is this environment familiar or unfamiliar? Is it loud? Quiet? What are the tonal qualities of the sounds around you? What are the scents? How does your body feel in this environment? Ask yourself what you need as you explore these questions. You have the power to leave if you do not feel safe.

When you are aware of what is occurring and how it's affecting your nervous system, you can respond to your needs. The following is an example of a client who knew what was happening physiologically when she became unsafe and was able to shift her own system back into safe engagement.

Candi's Story: A Client Who Uses Her Markers

Candi walked into my office twenty minutes late for her session. We had worked together for years, and I knew this was out of the norm for her since she was always on time.

She was pale and shaking. She plopped down onto the couch and just stared at the floor for several minutes. Because she was trauma informed, she knew she was dissociated. I kept my voice even and calm, assuring her to take her time.

"I'm right here," I said. "You're safe."

"Can I have the peppermint?"

She was referring to the essential oil I keep on my bookshelf. I handed her the bottle. Peppermint was a calming, grounding scent for her. It meant baking with her grandmother and all the times she felt loved and safe. It also happened to be stimulating enough for her olfactory senses to keep her out of dorsal vagal shutdown in past processing of traumas.

After sniffing the oil for a while, the color returned to her cheeks. She then said, "I got into an accident on the way over here. I was sitting at the light, and this dude slammed into me from behind. He totally wrecked my trunk, but I can still drive the car. It was unreal."

When she was five, Candi had been in a car accident in which her mother, who was driving, died. After this, she would kick and scream and run away if a grown-up tried to get her into a vehicle. For a while, the adults in her life understood and avoided driving with her in the car. But modern life is not conducive to walking everywhere. Over time, she was "forced" into cars. When she was, she spent the ride in a dissociative state of deep sleep, or if she appeared awake, she was not in her body. The grown-ups thought she was fine because she was so quiet and still in the back seat. However, as she sat there, Candi's brain and central nervous system stormed with a sense of danger. She could no longer use the sympathetic branch of her vagus nerve to run or fight her way out of the car. Instead, being what she would describe as "pinned in," her young brain collapsed her into dorsal vagal shutdown. From then on out, Candi would ride in cars and be deeply dissociated. She refused to get her license when she became a teen.

Not driving got problematic since she was relying on others to take her to school and her job. That is when she came to me to work through the trauma of the accident. She had even been too dissociated in those early years to mourn the loss of her mother.

First, we worked to help her to understand what was happening in her body and why. I gave her trauma definitions, so she felt empowered and not "crazy." We worked with techniques to help her connect to her body and the space she was in. She learned about the vagus nerve and how it had functioned to keep her safe. She was able to connect to the energy in her chakras and understand the emotional context of her experience. We processed the trauma memories using Eye Movement Desensitization and Reprocessing (EMDR). Over time, Candi no longer felt emotionally flooded with a feeling of danger when there was none. She could hold the memory of the accident in her mind without feeling she was still in the accident. She was also able to feel the loss of her mother without detaching from the emotions.

This current fender bender was retraumatizing her. The difference was that she now had skills to process through it.

I leaned in to see if she was feeling safe enough to connect with her eyes yet. "What do you need?"

"Just a minute." She sniffed some more peppermint, started to gently rock, then said, "I guess I need to call my insurance company."

As she fidgeted and moved, I could see she had gone from dorsal vagal shutdown to engagement with her sympathetic nervous system. She talked. I nodded and listened. She stood up. I pushed my chair back to make room for her as she shook her arms. She described the prickly energy that was running through them now. "I'm coming back into my body." She tipped her head from one side, then the other, and said, "I bet my neck is gonna hurt tomorrow, but I'm okay."

"Yes," I said, "you're safe now."

"Holy crud." She sat back down and looked me in the eyes. "I'm okay aren't I?"

"Yeah," I smiled. "You are, aren't you?"

She leaned forward and rested her hand on her heart. "My body is all right. I can feel it." As she had learned from our work, she drew in a breath and slowly released it to engage the ventral vagus nerve.

"You drove here after the accident?"

She nodded, then a smile crept in. "Crazy, huh? I could actually do that." She dropped her hand to her stomach where her sacral chakra rests. This chakra is the energy of emotional connection to others. Candi had a working knowledge of the chakras and was able to identify the sensation presenting in them. "It aches for her. I miss her. I really missed her today."

"I bet you did."

Tears welled in Candi's eyes. She sat for a long time and cried. I felt my own heart and sacral chakra open in this connection that was happening between us. I kept the space quiet and safe for her as she released her tears.

"It hurts," she said, tapping on her chest, "but I feel love here too."

Recapping the Three Branches of the Vagus Nerve

Let's do a quick recap to help you break down what you just learned about the three branches of the vagus nerve: the dorsal, the sympathetic, and the ventral vagal.

The dorsal vagal system activates by shutting you down when you are pinned in, unable to run or fight your way out of danger, have no options, or feel unimportant, unsupported, unheard, uncared for, neglected, or excluded from groups or people.

The sympathetic nervous system employs by stimulating fight or flight responses when you are threatened with physical or emotional harm, exposed to conflict or everyday stressors, feel pressured to perform, make choices, or meet deadlines, or indulge in unsafe narratives about yourself.

The ventral vagal system engages when you are connected to people you trust, feel centered within yourself, laugh or are calm, cuddle with safe people or pets, are connected to nature, or feel secure physically, emotionally, or psychologically.

Being aware of what is occurring in your body and identifying markers of safety is one way your vagus nerve can be supported. This is part of making friends with your body and seeing your nervous system as being in service of you.

EXERCISE
Writing Prompt: Getting to Know You

Write about a time you experienced a dorsal vagal state. What occurred? Do you remember the moment when it shifted? How did you feel in your body? Who was involved? What narratives about yourself or others did you have?

Write about a time you experienced a sympathetic state. What occurred? Do you remember the moment when it shifted? How did you feel in your body? Who was involved? What narratives about yourself or others did you have?

Write about a time you experienced ventral vagal safety. What did you feel in your body? How were you being with yourself and others? Where were you? What narratives about yourself or others did you have?

The Language of Body

There's a word that describes the sensations in your body and the meanings you apply to them based on the experiences that happen outside of you. That word is *interoception*. Once your interoception is understood, you can tend to your needs.[31] Consider this the sensing of emotions.

The client that I referenced earlier in this chapter, Candi, knew that that accident had dissociated her. She had reached for the oil that grounded and made her present. She breathed and stretched to help get her body to feel engaged again. She connected with another safe human. She let herself cry to release stress, and eventually, she felt the emotional engagement of missing her mother. She also let herself connect to those sensations in her sacral and heart chakras and identified the emotions that presented there.

You may be naturally attuned to the messages your body sends you and know how to tend to them. You may have developed coping mechanisms to push away anything you register as uncomfortable or overwhelming in your body. Perhaps you struggle with not knowing what is a trauma response versus an emotion. Having a vocabulary for personal experiences is important.

A term that Porges introduced with his polyvagal theory is *neuroception*.[32] While interoception is the awareness of what is occurring in your body, neuroception refers to how your nervous system responds to stimuli before you understand how your body responds to cues. It is the blink of eyes, the shift of a hand, the jerk of a torso, or the jumping at a loud sound.

---

31. Schwartz and Maiberger, *EMDR Therapy and Somatic Psychology*, 10.
32. Porges, "Emotion," 62–77.

The vagus nerve recruits your organs into the safety monitoring game. Your heart and the circulatory, respiratory, reproductive, digestive, and other systems send signals up to the brain. This is because you have visceral nerves that innervate these systems.[33]

Remember those times your stomach got upset when you missed a deadline? Or how your heart raced when your boss put more work on you? Those internal pains were not just your imagination. They were stress markers.

How about the tranquility you felt in your body when you held a loved one? When you are calm, safe, and connected, you experience ventral vagal responses in your whole body, including your organs. When you are feeling threatened or unsafe, those same organs are responding to your sympathetic arousal. This is called a visceral experience.

A visceral experience is different from a somatic one, but sometimes people use those words interchangeably. It may feel similar; however, somatic is felt through your skin, joints, tendons, ligaments, and fascia (the connective tissues).[34]

Do you remember a time when you felt an emotional sensation trickle over your skin? Have you ever experienced a fearful burn around your muscles? Perhaps you have gone to a doctor for a recurring back, neck, side, or other pain that they have not been able to diagnose? This may be an area of your body that is registering old emotional distresses. Where do you feel discomfort in your body when you are emotionally troubled?

Both your somatic and visceral nerve fibers send signals up to your brain via the main branches of the vagus nerve. Your brain then processes this information and sends "conclusions" back down

---

33. Netter, *Atlas of Human Anatomy*, 125.
34. Porges, *Polyvagal Safety*, 1–16.

the nervous system. This informational pattern is called bottom/up (body to brain) and top/down (brain to body) processing. It's important for you to observe what happens in your body because the visceral or somatic information is as important as the logical information your brain interprets. Much of your previously lived experience will drive the conclusions being made, which is the best argument for developing this awareness. It is a sensory experience that requires attuning.

EXERCISE
Mindful Walking

This exercise is intended to help you pay attention to your body differently. You walk every day to get to where you need to be, but how many times do you notice what you are feeling physically, emotionally, and psychologically while you are doing it? Walking is an amazing way for your central nervous system to find balance since the steps have a bilateral motion that engages both sides of your vagus nerve.

I would encourage you to walk outside, but if you can't, find a pathway in your home. When you walk, leave electronic devices behind. They are a great distraction for the central nervous system. Be mindful as you walk.

- As you breathe, notice the air. Is it warm? Cool? What do you smell? What does the air feel like in your lungs?
- Notice the colors and forms around you? Are these familiar locations? Look at the details of the trees, houses, cars, and sky in ways you may not have before.
- Allow any thoughts or judgments to arise, but don't follow them to conclusion. Thank the thoughts and focus back on your breath.

- Walk slowly and intentionally. Feel the sensations in your feet as you step. How do your legs feel? How do your limbs move?
- Be curious about what your body is doing. How do your clothes feel against your skin? What do your clothes sound like as they shift with your body?
- Take time to hear the sounds around you. Listen deeply without judgment. Are there noises in the distance that you have never heard before? Can you hear the sound of your breath?

Most people have been conditioned to believe all information is stored as a logical event, that the brain is your main source of news. However, your body holds some of the deepest knowledge you have. Accessing it requires listening differently because your body communicates in an implicit way. *Implicit* means you have memories unconsciously stored as neuronal pathways. The memories are felt. Your brain cannot pull from a visual or chronological recollection of an event. An example would be an experience as a baby that elicited an intense feeling. Maybe you got bitten by a dog when you were a year old, and now you have a mysterious fear of dogs. You implicitly carry that frightening memory in your nervous system.

Implicit memory is also responsible for procedural memory, such as tying shoes, buttoning shirts, running, or walking. It contributes to the motor skills you have developed through your life.

By being present to the sensations occurring in your body, you can communicate with yourself in a deeper way. Slowing down movement is one way to increase awareness of felt experience. Reminding yourself to check in with your body throughout the day is another. Notice your breath. Notice your posture. Be loving and curious.

Quite literally, trust your gut.

I mentioned implicit memory as presenting in your body. Explicit memories are those events, images, and scenarios that your brain holds. The triune brain, which I mentioned earlier, requires repetition for explicit memory to be stored. The multidimensional functions of the brain play various roles in this.

Remember those multiplication tables and alphabets you had to learn over and over again? How about those directions back to your house or another familiar place? Names, associations, or processes are all learned utilizing repetition and then stored in your brain for future needs. This requires going back over the information multiple times to develop explicit memories that create your exclusive reality in this life.

EXERCISE
Writing Prompt: From the Inside Out

This writing prompt might help you become more aware of the messaging in your body.

- Do you remember a time you had a visceral experience from your heart, stomach, or other organs? What was happening that caused the sensation? What did that feel like for you? This could be a racing heart because you're late or an upset stomach because a bill wasn't paid.

- Do you remember a time you had a somatic experience along your skin, joints, or the surface of your body? What was happening? What did a somatic experience feel like for you? This could be a nondescript back pain because of fear or a suddenly creaky neck because of an argument you had with a loved one.

Summary

You are so much more than what you can see. You possess a multilayered system that makes up your human existence. Those systems are both tangible and etheric. They construct your whole, and when you can recognize how they work in tandem and coordinate with each other, your authentic Self can utilize them for guidance. When you can access the more refined components of your messaging system, you make choices based on your authentic needs. Healing can become more profound and rapid when you're able to understand the psychophysiological is the spiritual and the spiritual is the psychophysiological. Both systems hold the connection to a peaceful future.

You have learned about your vagus nerve. Now let's look at your chakric system and how this felt experience can also act as a guiding principle for you.

CHAPTER 3
THE CONNECTION BETWEEN THE VAGUS NERVE AND CHAKRAS

•────────•

I n working with clients over the years, I have seen how their chakras parallel the emotional struggles they're healing. For instance, those who have ruptured connections to loved ones may feel the pain in their sacral and heart chakras. This is where the energy of relationships and love presents. Those who have been told their opinion didn't matter battle tightness in their throat chakra. Clients with eating disorders or addictive patterns report pain in the regions of their root or sacral chakras, which are the physical survival and relationship energies. Anyone with a strong need to control their world through overthinking seems to possess an intensity in their solar plexus and third eye chakras. They get headaches as they use the heavy charges of the solar plexus to shut down the intuitive qualities of the third eye.

The chakras exhibit both somatic and visceral responses. The energy of the chakras reaches deep within us as well as expands beyond our physical body. It is sending information as well as reading it. As these energy centers are connected to the vagus nerve, the messages are sent inward and travel through the organs, which we discussed is visceral, and through the fascia as somatic.

As examples, I have noticed clients feel both intestinal upset (solar plexus or sacral chakras/visceral) when processing loss of connection, as well as nondescript neck pain (throat chakra/somatic). They have also experienced openness in their throat (throat chakra/somatic) and release of tension along with an ability to breathe deeper (heart chakra/visceral).

Chakras are aligned with how the vagus nerve is delineated in your body. The lower three chakras (root, sacral, and solar plexus) connect to the unmyelinated (slower to move information) branches of the vagus nerve. The upper four chakras (heart, throat, third eye, and crown) connect to the myelinated (faster moving) branches, which are part of the ventral vagus, or social engagement, nerve branch. To date, there is no scientific research on the alignment of chakras and the vagus nerve. The information I am sharing with you comes from my professional observation of years of helping clients alleviate trauma responses and repair how they connected to others in childhood. As a student of Iyengar yoga, I have learned to work with chakras for my own psychospiritual balancing and that has naturally transferred over into the healing process.[35]

Based on these two foundations, I have paid attention to how my clients share their emotional and physiological responses during trauma processing, which is very mind- and body-centered processing. There is no doubt that these subtle energies are reflecting the personal experiences known to align with each psychological dimension of the chakras.

Many of my clients have very little, if any, reference to the chakras, which makes the expression of their emotional experience through the chakras more profound. At times, I don't even mention which chakra is presenting itself, as it takes them into their left-thinking brain and out of their present neurophysiological processing. However, it is helpful for me as I can see the emotional

---

35. B. K. S., *Light on Yoga*.

energy reprocessing in their system. The discussion of their chakras and the information they hold is often worked through later as we reflect on the session.

What Are Chakras

Chakras are etheric energy centers within your body. I like to say they need to be experienced more than seen. These rotating points of energy align with your torso and act like beacons that extend outward into the world and inward through the depths of your central nervous system, organs, and spine. Chakras are the unseen energies that make up your auric field and the "vibe" you give off as well as feel from others.

Like the vagus nerve, the chakras transport insights to and fro about how you're experiencing your reality. Unlike the vagus, I believe the essence of the chakras is Soul Self energy that is working in tandem with your human body—as if your Soul Self is driving the central nervous system like electricity runs a car's system.

There are known to be many chakric energy centers in the body, and the number depends on the branch of yoga a person studies. In this chapter, and throughout the book, I will focus on the seven chakras that line up with the torso and top of the head as I see these so cleanly aligning with the vagus nervous system. We also have energy centers within our hands and feet, and I will reference those as these contribute to your healing and the healing of others.

The awareness of chakras originated from the ancient practices of yoga and meditation.[36] The word *chakra* is Sanskrit for "wheel." Sanskrit is an ancient Indian language. Most Hindu scriptures are

---

36. Judith and Vega, *The Sevenfold Journey*, 6.

written in Sanskrit. Chakras reveal what ancient Hindu practitioners call prana. In simple terms, *prana* means the energy of life, or the breath of life, that flows through us.

This seven-chakra system comes from the branch of yoga in the *Purnananda* lineage, which may have begun around the 1500s. In the early twentieth century, Swiss psychoanalyst Carl Jung contributed to the normalization of chakras in Western psychology as a way for people to understand the more ethereic aspects of their psyche. He saw within these "psychic localizations" aspects of our consciousness. Jung felt chakras have within them the possibility of exploration and processing of your internal reality in a way that Western science was not open to.[37]

When overlaying ancient texts about the chakras and connecting them to modern scientific descriptions of the vagus nerve, you can utilize science and spirituality to a greater end. When chakras and the vagus nerve are looked at this way, deeper questions about your own healing and growth present themselves. Does your Soul Self utilize the nervous system as a "steering wheel" to engage energetically with the world? Are these experiences being generated up and down the fibrous branches of the vagus nerve to expand the Soul Self's understanding of being human?

The work of the Newton Institute, which studies what our Soul experiences between incarnations, has documented thousands of cases to show how the Soul enters the body and fuels its life force.[38] Founder Michael Newton, through his qualitative research, describes the chakras as a network of vital power points connecting to an ionized energy field flowing around our physical bodies (the aura).

---

37. Jung, *The Psychology of Kundalini Yoga*.
38. Newton, *Journey of Souls*, 97.

Kirlian photography, a type of film photography that has captured the colorful energetic field around us, has confirmed this.

Energy worker Donna Eden, in her seminal book *Energy Medicine*, experiences the chakras as circulating both clockwise and counterclockwise. She states she sees the chakras as possessing at least seven layers within them. Eden reports seeing multiple colors throughout each chakra when she is working with clients. An individual's chakras, she writes, "possess their own designs and are as unique to the person as their eye patterns or thumb prints."[39]

Dimensions of You

Just like your body needs tending, an awareness of your chakric health is important, particularly as it aligns with your vagus nervous system. Yoga, gentle movement, meditation, breath awareness, and mindful compassion are ways to keep these energy centers flowing.[40] Many of the exercises in this book will help facilitate this. These exercises have also been shown to engage and balance the social engagement branch of your vagus nerve. My intention is to have you understand these informational power centers and how they work for your body. Along with the vagus nerve, chakras are dimensions that make up your human self. They just possess more spiritual nature. Your journey through the chakras connects to your physical, emotional, psychological, and—eventually—spiritual you.

Physical, in this case, means the energy you carry in your body as a result of your experiences. As you read in the previous two chapters, your vagus nerve plays a huge role in this. What happens emotionally imprints physically. Painful events—but also love, kindness,

---

39. Eden, *Energy Medicine*, 147–59.
40. Porges, *Polyvagal Safety*, 89.
   Sullivan et al., "Yoga Therapy and Polyvagal Therapy," 88.

and support—are stored as information to be called upon at later times.

Emotional is the energetic experience that presents in the body utilizing the vagus nerve and the chakras. When you can be present to it, its complexity is astounding. My client Candi was able to feel the sadness of her loss, the fear from her accident, and the warmth of love for her mother through her chakras because she learned to not fear and to trust what her emotions were expressing through her body.

Psychological refers to the identities and adaptive behaviors you have acquired in this lifetime. Your persona with each experience you engage in, along with how you play out those roles in the world, is psychological.[41] We are all multidimensional in our identities and act them out with each circumstance.

Spiritual is the Soul or authentic Self. How easily your Soul can express in your body depends on how overpowering your psychological defenses are. The more you maneuver in the world with coping strategies that derived from emotional pain and the avoidance of it, the harder it is for your Soul energy to lead. When you heal childhood wounds, many of these obstacles dissolve. Your chakric energy then flows and your vagus nervous system is adaptable, which means your body can easily work its communication system.

Your Soul has a longing to expand and know. Because it is eternal, it has no fear. This is in direct contrast to our physical self, which wants to live at all costs and would kill or destroy another in service of physical survival. A balancing between these dichotomies takes a lifelong awareness and kindness to yourself.

---

41. Schwartz and Sweezy, *Internal Family Systems Therapy.*

EXERCISE
Breathing in Self-Compassion

Let's take a minute for you to connect to your body. This is a simple breathing and grounding technique to help you feel centered. When you feel centered, you feel loved because you feel safe.

- Put a hand over your heart and allow yourself to feel the palm-to-heart connection for a few seconds.
- Experience the comfort of your touch. Let this sensation ground you.
- Draw in your breath as you normally would and feel how the air fills your lungs. Sense that expansion within your upper rib cage.
- Continue to slowly draw your breath all the way into your torso.
- Allow the energy from your heart to spread across your chest.
- Repeat to yourself, "I am safe."
- What are you noticing?

The Sacred Seven

The seven major chakras in your system run from the top of your head, along the middle of your torso, and down to your pelvis. As you understand the qualities of the chakras and how they make up the dimensions of your human existence, you can utilize these energy centers with your vagus nerve for even more effective balancing.

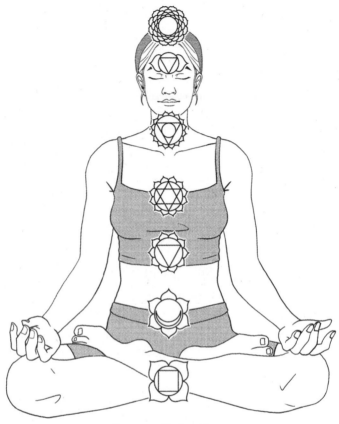

Figure 2: Chakra Figure

I call the chakras in the lower portion of the torso the "essential chakras." This has been my way of classifying as I work with clients. In this case, *lower* does not mean "less than." It simply means the chakras are present in the bottom portions of your torso and represent the deeper connections to your physical self, which connects to the physical world. Just like the sympathetic and dorsal vagal nerves are meant to help you engage in the very human ways that keep your body safe, the root, sacral, and solar plexus chakras ground you to your tangible reality.

The upper four chakras (heart, throat, third eye, and crown) connect to ventral vagus branches. I have coined these upper energy centers the "evolving chakras" because they invite you deeper into the connection of your inner world. When you reach inward, life becomes more symbolic, mysterious, and intuitive. These energy centers ask you to understand yourself in a nonlinear way.

Ventral vagal quality is what you need to anchor back into feeling safe and connected to your life.[42] This is where we have the space for engagement with our Soul. However, we need to have the adaptability in our nervous system to know when to read safety cues properly through the sympathetic and dorsal branches, always circling back around to ventral calm. It is a similar dynamic with the chakras. Utilizing the evolving chakras is an experience of tranquility, but the messaging of the essential chakras is also vital.

The Essential Chakras

When I am working with a client, the essential chakras are where I notice the hurt child aspects of them lay dormant. In other words, our "inner children" and their experiences become implanted in our systems here. These chakras were the first to develop in utero and infancy and speak to our primal needs of food and safety. If we did not get those needs met well, we hold those memories in our body. Fear, longing, and other uncomfortable emotions then present in your abdominal region where these chakras are. This is also where we get our bodily cues of hunger, sexual desire, physical connection, and need for shelter.

---

42. Dana, *Anchored*, 6.

The essential chakras are connected to the vagal neuronal fibers at the mid and lower regions of your diaphragm. Those nerves connect to the organs below the heart. These organs have no respiratory rhythm and are not autonomic in nature. The liver, spleen, and digestive system make up this region of your body. These chakra centers, like this area of the vagus nerve, are visceral. We can feel the intensity of the message from the inside out. Intensity, in this case, can be either pleasant or unpleasant feeling tones. Holding your lover can be felt just as strongly in this region of your body as being late for a job interview.

We need our basic requirements met before we can engage healthfully in other ways. We need to know how to manage our resources, connections to others, and our thoughts and boundaries to create safety in our world. When we are feeling uncertain about our ability to provide for ourselves (root) or unable to achieve and maintain healthy connections to others (sacral), our identity in the world is skewed (solar plexus). This is how I see aspects of essential chakras reveal themselves in sessions.

Body—The Root Chakra

The first chakra reveals the physical aspects of you. This chakra is the energy center related to bodily needs, including connection to the earth, food, shelter, resources, and survival. The root chakra is a reflection of physical safety. This chakra is located in the pelvis and is closest to the ground. I see this chakra engaged in regard to sexual activity as well, and when a client has been sexually violated, this chakric energy can get distorted.

Emotion—The Sacral Chakra

The second chakra connects us emotionally to others. The quality of your attachments reflects how safe you feel, which, of course, indicates how well you shape relationships of all kinds. The sacral chakra is a reflection of emotional safety. This chakra is located near the belly button, where the umbilical cord connected us to our first experience of life and safety.

Mind—The Solar Plexus Chakra

The third chakra charges you into action. It forms your sense of identity, ego, and personality, which is shaped through concepts of your mind and how you see reality. The solar plexus bridges you from the experience of your basic needs into an awareness of your world and how you fit into it. This chakra is located in the sternum at the crux of the ribcage.

The Evolving Chakras

The evolving chakras begin the journey into deeper awareness and personal meaning. These chakras are the avenue to your Soul Self. This energy brings you into your authenticity. The energy in these chakras is connected to the vagus nerve that originates in the brain stem and travels to the organs above your diaphragm. These organs are part of your autonomic nervous system. The nerves in this area of your body are coated (myelinated), which means information travels faster along these fibers for rapid processing. Very similar to how intuitive knowing seems to just show up.

The heart chakra is the energy that expands beyond the organs of the heart and lungs. The heart, and its heart rate, with the help of the breath, is what determines how well a person can manage and stabilize their "vagal brake" or emotional safety system with their breathing.

The throat chakra is connected to the nerve fibers that support the larynx, jaw, tongue, middle ear, and face. This region of ventral vagal nerve endings is helping you interact with others through speech, hearing, and physical sight. The throat chakra is the energy of relatedness and, in this case, is more complex than just the tones we express. With the assistance of the vagal nerve fibers, this chakra extends beyond the region of your larynx and flows into the mouth and ears.

The third eye chakra connects to the sinuses, thalamus, hypothalamus, and pituitary gland, which helps maintain hormonal balance and peace within the brain and nervous system. It also is placed before the prefrontal lobe, which is our place of higher reasoning. Through this chakra, you connect to the unspoken language of symbol, energy, and color, which is the language of the Soul Self.

The crown chakra rests on the top your head, at the crux of your prefrontal cortex, where your soft spot as an infant was. This chakra acts like an open receiver of spiritual information from the higher realms. The energy filters down to the higher reasoning brain, the midbrain, and throughout the central nervous system.

All the qualities of the evolving chakras allow for inner awareness and spiritual growth. Below, I have broken down the qualities of these chakras as I have seen them show up in sessions.

Intuition—The Heart Chakra
The fourth chakra directs you to a deeper relationship with your Soul Self. When you can "drop down" into you, your sense of knowing expands. Your love for yourself and others increases as this energy is soothing and safe. This chakra is located in the chest in the area of your heart.

Connection—The Throat Chakra
The fifth chakra allows you to manifest your creative power by speaking your truth and hearing the truth of others. When this energy

center is flowing, you can ask for what you need and convey concepts. This energy, more than any other chakra center, creates and invites healing tones and sounds. This chakra is located in the throat.

Spirituality—The Third Eye Chakra

The sixth chakra leads you into your subjective Soul Self. It is the access point to your unique symbolism, energy, and internal information. This chakra connects you to that which makes up your inner world. Trusting its symbolic communication helps you to trust that not all things spiritual can be discerned using a linear process. This chakra is located between the brows.

Empathy—The Crown Chakra

The seventh chakra connects you to the greater universe. It is webbing to all that exists. When we attach to the higher realms, we begin to understand we are all part of a network of humanity, which deepens our understanding and compassion. This chakra is located in the middle front of the skull.

EXERCISE

What If There Were No Words?

You interact from your intuitive and biological selves every day—with or without words. You are using an intricate system of neuronal patterns in your brain, central nervous system, muscles, fascia, and your chakras. All of this is fueled by your interpretations and intentions. Some of this comes from so deep inside of you that before you make meaning out of it, you have an internal response (nueroception). It is a universal language that people are both sending and receiving. When we are disconnected from our responses to stimuli, our outcomes reflect this. When we are mindfully attuned to our body's physiological responses, how we connect with others will be different, and this will reflect in our relationships.

Imagine, for a moment, a world with no words. No written way to communicate. No ability to frame concepts with the language you know.

How would you connect with others? How would you share ideas, feelings, experiences, and the realities of your mind? Your concepts would be unlike anything you could currently imagine. Without the words and numbers that built its infrastructures, society would not look as you know it.

- Be still for a minute and ask yourself how you would communicate without words. For a deeper understanding of what this would feel like, sit on your hands. Let yourself experience how you would connect with the people around you. What do you notice? How do you understand your body right now?

- Track the feeling state in your body as you imagine approaching someone you know and love. How would you be? Where do you feel emotional currents within you? Is there a sense of expansion? Contraction? Flow? Sit with yourself for a while and notice.

- Imagine yourself approaching someone you don't trust. Continue tracking the sensations in your body. Notice your breathing and any tension in your system—both inside and out. Where do you feel tightening? What is the difference between this visualization and the previous exercise? How are you understanding your body's emotional responses?

Let's keep going with this visualization.

- Shift the scene and see yourself approaching a stranger, a neutral party. Maybe you know them, maybe you don't. This person is somewhere on the periphery of your life. What does your body feel now?

One more visualization.

- See a baby wrapped in a soft blanket, smelling like freshness. Breathe in and get closer to the image. See the baby's face and gestures. This child is connecting in the only way it knows how, and you are responding in turn. In what ways are you experiencing the communication? What's going on in your system? So much of your response might have to do with how you interpret infants to begin with. Is this image of a baby you love?

EXERCISE
Writing Prompt: The Emotional Is the Physical

Of the four people that you engaged with in your mind's eye, which felt pleasant in your body? Which felt unpleasant or neutral? What did you notice that changed with each visualization, and where did you feel it? What were the sensations? Was it through the muscles and skin that your body responded? Did you feel things deeper within yourself through your stomach or other organs? Where? What surprised you the most?

If you are a visual processor, use your colored pencils to draw where in your body you felt these experiences.

Trust the Experience

If you have never worked with your chakras before, it may take time to feel their flow, especially if you habitually dissociate from your body. Once you connect, you might still be uncertain as to what you're experiencing. Just take it slow. Heighten your awareness. Use the exercises in this book to draw attention to your body through your vagus nerve and chakras. Be curious and kind. This will lead to a loving connection to yourself.

If chakra work, through yoga or other practices, is something you do regularly, then I invite you to deepen your psychological connection to them by understanding this energy reaches deep within your system. Notice how you experience emotions in your body. Be intrigued and open to a greater engagement. Be an observer of yourself as you participate in the world and with others.

While there is a framework regarding energetic systems, such as the chakras, being present to their energy is a unique experience. It's exclusive to you. There is no right or wrong when you are honoring how you are feeling. Right or wrong are by-products of our brain needing to make sense, and some things need to just be experienced without outcome. Tuning into your body's energy is ineffable. Words can be limiting.

Just breathe and trust this new way of being. Over time, this way of tuning into yourself and interacting with the world will be second nature.

Hierarchy of Needs in Relation to the Chakras

The chakras are heralds, echoing your innermost realities outward and revealing your personal truths. Each reflects the dimensions of your human needs. When you follow the chakras upward, from the physical to the spiritual, you can see this.

The humanist Abraham Maslow established five levels of needs that humans possess and strive for.[43] It has been coined as "Maslow's Hierarchy of Needs." You may have seen this displayed as a pyramid since many people have taken his words and put them into graphic form.

The first of these needs are basic physiological ones, such as food, air, and places to extricate bodily waste. According to Maslow, you cannot exist without tending to your body first. This is also the energy of the root chakra. We cannot engage in our human experience if we don't manage ourselves physically.

Maslow then asserted that people seek safety and security by creating resources for themselves. Through shelter or monetary exchanges, we secure our health. This solidifies our physiological needs. Once these needs have been met, Maslow hypothesized, humans reach outward for social connection, love, and friendship (which is still a safety need through the polyvagal perspective). This is the connection we seek through the energy of the sacral chakra.

Being in relationships with others and the identity we have in our community is reflected in solar plexus energy. This mirrors Maslow's fourth need: desire for self-esteem, social status, or mastery of a craft or profession as ways to achieve recognition. The energy in the solar plexus mirrors the dimension of mind.

These above four needs were coined as deficiency needs. What Maslow referred to as biology, connection, or power needs, I see as essential chakra needs. These essential chakras help establish us before we even make our way into adulthood.

As a person obtains levels of security in the world, they now have the means and time to reach inward to explore who they are. This brings us into the evolving energy of the heart and intuitive

---

43. Maslow, "'Higher' and 'Lower' Needs."

energy of the throat chakras. The imaginal aspects of the third eye, and, certainly, the crown chakra of connection carry us upwards into a higher realm. Maslow wrote that we are all working toward self-actualization. This is where the experience of the evolving chakras and the ventral vagal branch of safety meet.

As you follow and learn about the chakras in part 2 of the book, notice how your needs mirror this order.

PART 2
HEALING THROUGH
THE CHAKRAS AND
THE VAGUS NERVE

CHAPTER 4
BODY AND THE ROOT CHAKRA

————•————

The root chakra places you firmly on the ground and gives you the earthly awareness your Soul Self has been seeking.[44] This chakra regulates the physical dimensions of being human. It connects you to resources, safety, sexual function, and food. Located in the pelvis, this energy is associated with surviving but also thriving. The root chakra is associated with the color red. Red—the color of blood. It doesn't get more tangible and human than that.

Like the roots of a plant, this chakra asks you to reach deep into the ground to receive nourishment. Nourishment, in this case, is a steady grounding and engagement with the physical aspects of yourself. How you are being in your body is how your Soul Self is experiencing this world.

Through the body, you experience the tangy sweet of an orange, the cool scent of wet pine trees along the northern coast, the warm smoothness of a cat's purring belly, and the angelic wetness of a baby's kiss on your face. Without the body, your Soul Self cannot know the pleasure of these things.

Your body holds early life experiences that even your brain cannot promptly access. Your body is psychic. It feels deep emotions, intuits other realms, and feels a knowing for the unquantifiable.

---

44. Johari, *Chakras*, 85.

In this way, the root chakra, while sometimes brushed off as basic, is one of the most spiritual chakras you possess.

One more note on grounding: the work we are doing and my references about it do not exclusively apply to a physical grounding. The root chakra will emotionally ground you in safety as you become more comfortable with what it's trying to tell you. The biggest take-away I hope you get from this book is to befriend your physical self and understand it works as a spiritual compass for you.

EXERCISE
Body Scan

I want you to employ a technique you can return to time and again called the body scan. The body scan stems from mindfulness meditation, which is a Buddhist practice. It's intended to help you deepen your spatial awareness, increase the messaging in your body, and connect to your breath and feeling states.

Breathing is something we do from the autonomic portion of our nervous system. In other words, we don't even think about it. Breathing just happens. However, when we can pull in breaths with awareness, we can develop a sense of our own physical space and how we are in it.[45]

- To start, find a comfortable chair to sit in. As you settle, locate your bones so that you have alignment but not tension in your spine. Be aware of the sensation of your hips in the seat. How do your back and arms feel in the chair?
- As you become aware of your presence in the chair, know that you are safe.

---

45. Kabbat-Zinn, *Full Catastrophe Living*, 75.

- Now draw your attention to the top of your skull. Just notice. Be curious. What are the sensations? Is there tension? Warmth? Coolness?

- Bring your focus downward to your forehead, your ears, your jawline. What do you become aware of? How do the muscles feel? If need be, pull a breath into this area of your body.

- Continue down to your neck, throat, and shoulders. Stay curious. As you anchor your awareness to this area of your body, note the sensations.

- Imagine your breath filling this area of your body. Notice.

- When you're ready, scan down between your shoulder blades, chest, and arms. This is the area of your lungs. What does the breathing feel like here? Where in your lungs do the breaths connect before they are released?

- Travel your attention down to the torso and diaphragm. Notice how the muscles are held. How are you placed in the chair? Where is tension? Be curious. Notice if any judgment arises. Be gentle and then let it float outside of you, accepting that it's there but not taking it in.

- Shift attention down to your hips, lower back, and pelvis. This is an area of your body that puts in a lot of work. What senses arise? Be present to them. Pull in a few breaths, and imagine the oxygen as nourishment to the muscles.

- After a while, notice your thighs and knees. Any aches or pains? Just be aware without attempting to change anything. What is tense? What is relaxed? Imagine the breaths going downward.

- Continue to be curious as you draw attention to your ankles and feet. What do you notice. Just breathe.
- As you lean into your full body awareness, notice beliefs or thoughts. Do you want to avoid any aspects of your body? Do you want to fix anything? Don't respond. Just notice and stay kind and curious. Even if judgmental thoughts arise, see them as if evolving from a place beyond yourself while still being very present to yourself. Utilize the language of "there is judgment" or "there is tension" or "there is calm."

Being fully present to the moment makes you a conscious observer in your own life. We become so conditioned to rush in and fix when we perceive the slightest discomfort that it doesn't occur to us to just stay curious. Stay lovingly present to your body for as long as you need during these scans. Do this technique daily if you want. The more you become aware of how your body feels, the gentler you will be with yourself.

The Vagus Nerve and the Root Chakra

The vagus nerve fibers that link up with your root chakra connect to your lower abdomen and lumbar region of your back (coccygeal spinal ganglion). These fibers attach to the colon, the small intestines, ascending colon, sexual organs, and even the appendix. Hormonally, the hypothalamic-pituitary-gonadal (HPG) axis acts in concert with these organs. The hormones secreted from the HPG axis play a big part in regulating your reproductive and immune systems.[46]

---

46. Netter, *Atlas of Human Anatomy*, 125.

Can you see how, if you are in a constant state of fear, your system gets compromised over time? Your lower intestines may release waste too frequently when you perceive a threat or hold on to excrement. Discomfort in this area of your body can lead to over- or undereating because your physical signals are crossed. Stress can change menstrual cycles and the ability to obtain or maintain an erection. Your root chakra can employ sensations of intensity, pain, and sexual overdrive or underfunctioning when the body is on high alert.

As mentioned, our organs respond based on memories of safety—or lack thereof—because they are connected to the vagus nerve.[47] As a result, the organs can inspire visceral responses that show up as unpleasant feeling tones. As counterintuitive as this sounds, this is a wonderful opportunity for you to embrace the experience and be open to the messages your body, in its state of distress, is telling you. Remember, bodily discomfort when there is no impending doom can provide an important mapping system to the things we need to heal from in our past.

This process is an effort to keep us alive. So, why wouldn't this reveal itself in the subtle energies of the root chakra? The Soul is here to dance on the earth. The Soul feels and experiences what the body is communicating. Are you prone to intestinal issues when you worry about money? Do you suffer back pain when your job gets stressful? As you become more attuned to this root chakra, you will also be able to identify psychological messages through this energy center.

When we feel secure and calm, these organs also link with ventral vagal fibers and create more neutral or pleasant feeling

---

47. Porges, *The Polyvagal Theory*, 54.

tones.[48] When we experience calm, the organs in this area, near our pelvis, hips, and lower back, go about their jobs with us hardly noticing (neutral feeling tones).

Let's get to know and connect to the root chakra and develop awareness of our vagus nerve in this area of our body. Feeling grounded with your legs and feet is an important place to start. These subtle and physical energies are reciprocal.

Chandelar's Story: Disconnecting from Emotions Means Disconnecting from the Body

Chandelar came to me because he was having a hard time focusing at work. He said he liked to "work things out in his head," but lately this way of seeking solutions was getting tougher.

We went through his family history. Chandelar reported no childhood trauma and described a very good relationship with his parents. He was the youngest child of three and the only boy. Both sisters live in the same small town with his parents and care for them as they age. Chandelar said he was the only one in the family who ever lived outside of the small town. His move for work as a mathematics professor had brought him to the other side of the country. He told me he didn't get home regularly because of this. He also said he was a hundred pounds overweight but felt that was genetics since he didn't snack between meals.

As our work deepened and I got to know Chandelar's lifestyle, it became apparent he would binge drink or heavily smoke pot when he was socializing. He consumed so severely that he found himself passing out at parties or waking up on strangers' sofas. His drinking and pot smoking patterns did not fit addiction criteria. He

---

48. Porges and Dana, *Clinical Applications of the Polyvagal Theory*, 106–24.

didn't crave or imbibe in either unless he was out with friends. It was obvious that he was using these numbing tactics to calm social nerves and couldn't decipher his own limits.

Each session, with no prompting from me, he would shift between complaining about his weight to stating he was fine with it. He'd been dating the same woman for two years, but he didn't want to get too serious—despite the fact that she did. He said he liked to keep people "at bay." He told me he would spend a lot of time reading or binge-watching television. When we discussed anyone close to him, he would look away or change the subject.

Helping Chandelar connect to his emotional world through identifying feelings in his body was a slow go. It took months of weekly sessions and him learning to trust me as well as the process. First, we started to connect the dots between the experiences he had with others and his behaviors. He noticed how he would binge-watch television for hours following conversations with his parents. He saw how he reread the same sci-fi novels from childhood each time he got off work and didn't have anything to do. Over time, he was able to recognize his social media scrolling patterns when he was supposed to be working. One day he came in with a diary of his food intake.

"I thought you might want to see this." He handed me a notebook. "You know how I like to make lists. It's everything I ate for the last month."

I glanced through it. I am not a registered dietitian, so I don't supervise what foods my clients consume, even when we are directly working on an eating disorder. My work is not to help manage another's behaviors. I help clients identify actions that are harmful, explore why and how they engage in those actions, and utilize ways to help them heal from dynamics that no longer serve them.

"I mean," he put his hands up, "I might not eat between meals but look at what I'm eating!"

"Yep," I said and handed him back the notebook. "That's a lot of food."

"I'm numbing with that, too, huh?" He was starting to learn the difference between dissociating from perceived threats versus self-care or "down time."

I nodded. "It's really good you're recognizing this." I smiled and leaned in. "Now, wanna explore it deeper?"

He laughed. "You're not gonna take away my ice cream sandwiches, are you?"

"Promise," I said. "First step of the mapping system complete. You're seeing the 'what.' Now let's get to the 'why' so we can discover the 'where' and 'how.'"

"Why, where, and how?" he asked.

"Why you are numbing. Where you are feeling it in your body, and how to look curiously at it."

Something in Chandelar lit up from this point forward. He was ready to understand why he wanted to shut down and dissociate so frequently now that he knew he was doing it.

We revisited his family dynamics. His biggest fear was that we would be betraying his parents if he shared any stories they perceived as negative. Once he understood family patterns form how we engage in the world—and there are just as many "good" as "bad"—he readily explored his childhood. He noticed how his parents and sisters "numbed" when they felt overwhelmed.

"It's kind of a collective," he said. "They have these humongous meals together several times a week. Then they all sit around and watch a movie until Dad falls asleep. After these meals, I would always go off to my room and read." Chandelar shook his head.

"I felt guilty at how much I hated those times. It was," he took in a deep breath, "suffocating."

Chandelar started to understand his family's subtle messaging that outside the house was scary and inside was safe. However, inside never allowed him his own boundaries or interests. His parents expected Chandelar to take part in everything they did and told him no one outside the family would be as good to him as they were. His family's insistence that he "be like them" forced Chandelar to detach from his own wants and needs just to be in relationships with the people he loved.

When he got the professorial job at a university across the country, it was an acceptable way to leave. However, aspects of Chandelar never left home. He took his beliefs and coping strategies with him. Each time he engaged socially, his nervous system screamed that he was unsafe, and he shut it down with the depressants of pot and alcohol. When he was alone, he was uncertain as to what he wanted or needed, so he escaped into his favorite books from childhood. He numbed his anxiety until he couldn't feel anything physically or emotionally. This led to depression and further separation from his inner world. Chandelar was under the notion that anxiety was actual emotion and not physiological responses generated by the way he thought. Once he understood that even what he labeled as a difficult emotion—sadness, anger, fear—had a soft capacity to guide him, he made room for it. He became less apt to engage in behaviors that shut himself down because he was learning to trust this inner guidance.

As he made friends with his body, we were able to help him identify where the fearful childhood messages were stored. I was using an approach with Chandelar called Internal Family Systems

(IFS) therapy that helps a client identify aspects of their childhood selves that may carry old belief systems and coping strategies.[49]

Discomfort always presented deeply in his lower abdomen at his root chakra. He misinterpreted feeling this fear as hunger cues, which was the reason for his heavy meals. As he learned to be present to his somatic uneasiness without attempting to escape from it, he was able to listen to what his body was saying.

"My stomach feels upset, but it always feels like this." He placed his hand on his lower abdomen. "I'm not gonna get sick."

"Can you breathe deeper into it? Be gentle and curious."

After a while, Chandelar said, "I suddenly have this memory of my dad coming home after losing one of his many jobs. I was probably six. He called us all into the living room and told us his boss was stupid, and it wasn't his fault he got fired. He said we had to stick together and cut back on things. That we couldn't trust anyone outside of the family." Chandelar opened his eyes and looked over at me with a grimace. "My father lost a lot of jobs, and it was always because of a 'stupid' boss."

"How did that six-year-old you experience this?"

He closed his eyes again and pulled in a deep breath. "I was scared. I was mad at my dad's boss. I felt helpless and worried about all of us." He paused. "But I also felt angry. Why did we have to know this? What could I have done? I was just a kid. I was so overwhelmed, I went to sleep for hours after that."

"How do you feel toward this child?"

"I feel—worried for him." Chadelar put his hand on his stomach.

"Does this younger you know he is in an adult body now?"

---

49. McConnell, *Somatic Internal Family Systems Therapy*, 25.

Chandelar kept his eyes closed and was silent for a while. "He does now. He sees me."

"What is he experiencing as he sees you?"

"Relief."

"Can you ask him what he needs from you?" I said.

"A hug," he kept his eyes closed. "He just wants to be on his skateboard and not worry about Dad or if there's gonna be food in our house to eat."

"Does he want you to skate with him?"

"Yes." Chandelar was silent for a long time but deeply connected to what was happening internally. "I'm telling him I take care of the bills now. He doesn't have to worry. God knows, we have plenty to eat! This makes him happy." He opened his eyes. "He just jumped on the board and rode off. He's happy."

"Check in with that root chakra we talked about earlier," I said. "What do you notice?"

"Pain is gone," he said. "This area of my body is calmer than I've ever felt it."

Following this experience, I led Chandelar through some deep breathing that connected to his lower abdomen and root chakra. The deeper he trusts this area of his body and its messages, the more he will be able to honor his safety needs.

Deepening Your Roots

I have mentioned the seven major chakras; however, there are two other energy centers that are so intertwined with the root chakra we need to get to know them.

Feet

The first is the pair of chakras in your feet. Being aware of and utilizing this energy will help you. It simply takes awareness.

Your feet are probably the most used yet most neglected part of your body. Think of what you do with them. We run or walk for miles or don't walk on them at all. We neglect their care and take for granted that those small bones, tendons, and muscles will always carry us where we want to go.

When we dissociate from our bodies through lack of movement and numbing, we start to walk less over time. When we dismiss the importance of our feet, they atrophy through edema and bloating. More weight than our bodies need appears, and it gets harder to move.

When you are walking or meditating outside, open up these centers. Pull in earth energy—the best kind of grounding energy there is. Bringing attention to this area of your body is important, and knowing we have this chakra center in our arches will help you with a sense of balance.

Hara

The second energy system is the hara. This energy appears above the root chakra and just beneath the sacral chakra. If you soften your belly, you might feel an "extra" source of energy in this area. The more I personally draw attention to mine, the more physically balanced and grounded I feel myself to be.

The hara seems to hold a combination of both the root and sacral chakra qualities.[50] The energy of emotional safety feels strong in this area. It's the will to live, thrive, protect, defend, and connect.

The hara, which is the Japanese term for this energy center, is not discussed often. It seems to come online more frequently as my clients start to heal from early childhood traumas and are

---

50. Abbate, *The Hara, the Source of Life and the Navel, the Gate of Spirit.*

able to stay more connected to their body. I have seen this with clients and have had personal observation and experience as well. I call this the spiritual warrior chakra. It at once seeks power and gentleness.

Like all the chakras, this one can be connected with through mindful attention in meditation, yoga, or purposeful movement, such as walking. For me, I find my hara feels in sync when I engage in faster bilateral movement such as hiking or cycling. I cycle and that movement helps me feel more energetically connected to the lower portion of my body. You don't need a bike to engage with any of these energy centers. Gentle squats or standing poses in yoga activate this region. As always, be gentle and just notice.

EXERCISE
Get Grounded

This is a simple exercise I had Chandelar do to help him understand the concepts of grounding and feeling connection to his body. All it takes is some intention and a grassy, safe place to go barefoot in.

- Take any footwear off and look at your feet. You can stand or sit down as you do this. Say hello to your arches, toes, and ankles. Wiggle your toes and spread them as wide as you can.
- What does it feel like to move your toes? Have you ever looked closely at your feet?
- Keeping your heels on the ground, lift the balls of your feet upward to get a full stretch. Stay like this for as long as you can without too much strain. Notice where you experience tightness or tension. What do

your ankles feel? What other muscles are you using to stretch? Stay present to this for a while.

- Now, spread your toes as wide as they will go as you aim them toward the ceiling. What do you sense? If you get tired, rest the balls of your feet back on the ground.

- Pressing the balls of your feet on the ground, lift your heels. Keep spreading your toes. Let yourself sense the energy exchange through your legs. Be aware of all the different muscles that are working. Which ones are stretching versus which ones are actively lifting?

Have your feet and legs woken up? Is there more circulation in them? Your feet hold up a precious stronghold that helps you engage with your world. Thank your feet for all the hard work they do.

EXERCISE
Writing Prompt: Your Precious Stronghold

As you move your feet, draw attention to your legs and hips. Allow the new awakening in your legs and feet to extend to your pelvis. Notice any colors and textures around this area of your body. Draw these textures and colors in the way you are experiencing them.

Use words on the paper to describe what you feel. Are there subtle changes on how you connect to your body now? Is there resistance? What is your experience? What is different about the way your lower body feels?

Attunement: The Highest Expression of the Root Chakra

Attunement is the intention you bring to balancing your system and tending to your needs. It calls for you to be present to the moment so you can define those needs. When you attune to your body, a sense of self and your place in your world come more easily. Your body becomes your home and a haven. Whether you approach this from a polyvagal or chakra lens, being present is what helps you manage your physiological response.

Hold space and listen. Respect what your body is telling you. See it as your compass. The energetic flow both inside and outside of your body will guide you when you learn to listen to it. Through your body, you will then work more intuitively. When you catch yourself in a harsh dialogue about yourself or others and choose to redirect this, you can hear your authentic Self more clearly. Your body speaks a truth. It is your informational messaging center.

Part of attunement is to know when your nervous system and chakras are in appropriate sync with the present moment reality. Being gentle and responding in kindness is the way to honor our body. Self-care is not selfish.

No one will care for you better than you should care for yourself. No one will ever love you more than you should love yourself. You draw in a similar frequency that matches your own vibration. People can only love you on the same frequency that you are able to love yourself.

Healing happens over time. Nurturing and growth are a lifelong consciousness. Intention to heal needs to be developed and that requires trusting who you are in your present moment. Understand that with each level of growth comes a new one.

An incredible flow of energy works through you when you're doing things "right." Right is not what others think you need to be doing. Right is what you need to be doing, and the only way to be "right" is to attune to your own needs.

Control: The Lowest Expression of the Root Chakra

When you are locked in a narrative of "not enough," you work from a premise of wanting to control situations around you. When you feel a need to keep things the way you believe they should be, then your body constricts and engages too frequently with your sympathetic nervous system. That fight or flight response tightens muscles, increases blood pressure, and restricts your root chakra. You are not present to yourself because you are scanning for things to be the way you think you need them to be.

Whether you believe you have plenty or none, your perspective shapes your reality. "Not enough" puts you in a mindset of control over others.[51] A mindset of lacking creates tension with others because you see them as competition for resources. Controlling things you cannot really control is a misinformed belief that you can soothe yourself from the outside in.

This dance is done in a misled attempt to keep from feeling pain. Fearing the idea of pain leads to many heavy layers of protection, including refusing to believe you even feel fear. Ironically, denial creates so much more pain than it attempts to avoid. It allows harmful attachments to continue. It permits dangerous behaviors to escalate. It permits injury to self and others through passive-aggressive actions and words.

---

51. Evans, *Controlling People*, 10.

Like a ripple in a pond, the attempt to deny sends out negative consequences that affect people and families for years and generations.[52] When it's done in governments and businesses, it destroys lives and the planet. Fear is short served, but the outcome is long term. The only way to manage your world is from the inside out. When you trust your inner world, you can attune to yourself and leave others to their own path.

EXERCISE
Writing Prompt: What You Can and Can't Control

This is an exercise you can go back to regularly. It's especially helpful during those times when you feel things are chaotic or you have a big decision to make and are struggling with doing so. You can also do this when you want to explore your basic outlook on life. What can you control? What can't you control?

- In your journal, draw a line down the center of the paper. As a header on the left side of the line, write *CAN*. On the right header, write *CAN'T*.
- Now think of a situation in your life that is bothering you. In the CAN'T column, write all the things about this situation you cannot control. In the CAN column, write all the things in it you can control. Write everything you can think of for both sides of the columns. Continue writing until you have exhausted all thoughts about this.

What is in your CAN control column? What is in your CAN'T control column?

---

52. Menakem, *My Grandmother's Hands*, 179.

Know that whatever is in your CAN'T column you can let go of because the fact is, it's never been within your control to begin with. Those things in your CAN control column need to be tended to in a realistic manner.

The CAN'T control column can now bring space into your awareness. This is where you can now breathe more easily. Let it go. Let those that need to focus on their own responsibilities do it. Notice how your body feels as you understand that on a universal, emotional level these things have never been yours. Release them. Let them fly to their appropriate owners. Don't even worry about who owns them. They will find their way.

Enjoy the freedom and emotional space you can now experience in your body. Continue to just breathe and release by using any of the exercises you have already experienced in the previous chapters of this book. Breathe.

Recognizing Body Blocks

How you engage with your body is how you engage with your world. How do you feel about your body? How do you feel about your place in your world?

There is a tension involved in being physically aware of your emotional state. Your work comes in being able to acknowledge this, to accept tension is a part of life. Being uncertain to an outcome, no matter how large or small, is an example of holding tension. Even in meditation, tension is present. Holding your body upright enough to feel centered and connected is its own form of tension.

Messages get filtered outward—sometimes by well-meaning people—that say you are complete only when you are calm and blissful, that if you don't maintain this state of being you're not doing life properly. How can anyone live up to that expectation of themselves? The belief of "only happy" would require you to block all other messages and close off most of the information coming from your central nervous system or etheric energy. When this happens, you can only set yourself up for various states of detachment from your body. Some of the ways we disconnect are:

- Drugs and alcohol
- Binging or restricting food
- Sex, porn, or constantly pursing new relationships
- Excessive use of electronic devices, such as video games, television, or phones
- "Busy-ness" such as working too much, interacting on social media, overjoining organizations, talking out of nervousness, constantly seeking connection with others for fear of being alone, taking on too many responsibilities, overcleaning
- Overly focused on others by trying to worry about or control them
- Directly self-harming through cutting, picking, scraping skin, hair pulling, excessive exercise, and sports injuries
- Indirectly self-harming by allowing others to physically hurt you
- Negative talk about self or others
- Spiritual bypassing by excessive meditation or spiritual practices
- The overs—oversleeping, overexercising, overeating, etc.
- Raging to distract from more vulnerable emotions

Even if you are not engaging in risky or dangerous behaviors to avoid what you perceive as unwanted emotion, distractions from unpleasant feeling tones are still tempting. Knowing what you are feeling and when you are diverting yourself is key. That way you can understand what is occurring within you and reach for some loving ways to ground and care for yourself.

None of us can live a full, balanced, prosperous, loving, sensuous life if we're physically disconnected from it. The body is the core representation of your psychological and spiritual well-being. Befriending your body with intelligence and kindness is lifelong maintenance. If you have been told all your life that your body was not worthy or good enough, now is the time to move beyond those beliefs. Know that through your body you experience connection with your Soul.

So many cultures and religious beliefs see the body as an obstacle to overcome, a repulsive form that has to be isolated, shamed, and conformed. Have you spent decades rejecting and mutilating your body? Have you starved it just to be accepted and loved?

True healing from these messages is an unfolding and starts with an intention to know yourself better. Heal the past hurts within the safe containment of a licensed therapist's office. Utilize gentle movements of yoga, tai chi, or qigong, or simply walk. You will soon understand there is no monster in the shadows of your body as much as there is a screaming, scared child who is simply asking to be loved.

EXERCISE
Mindful Awareness of Your Root Chakra

Settle into the sacred space you have created and find a comfortable place for you to sit. If you want to light a fragrant candle or use essential oils, do so. The scents will activate your olfactory nerves and will induce ventral vagal activity. Remind yourself that you are in a comfortable, calm place.

- Notice how you feel sitting in your seat. Draw awareness to the pressure on your hips, lower back, legs, and other areas that connect to your chair. Soften your gaze or close your eyes. Pull some deep breaths into your lower abdomen.
- As you exhale, release the breath slowly as this engages ventral vagal activity.
- Then shift your attention deeper into to your pelvic area. What do you notice?
- Be curious about the energy arising, knowing this is an etheric extension of your vagus nervous system.
- Allow for the dual awareness of both your breathing and how your pelvis feels. The sensation of the root chakra should begin to emerge. What are you experiencing?

Addendum to this Exercise

If turning inward is a struggle, please be gentle with yourself. You may have had childhood experiences that forced you to be still when you wanted to run or fight, so being still recreates that experience for you. You are safe now.

I deeply encourage you to walk or stretch if sitting still is too fear provoking. Apply the same mindful attunement to your movement and just notice the energy around your pelvis. When anxiety arises, look around and remind yourself you are safe. Feel the ground beneath you. Let your feet connect to the texture of the ground. Continue to connect to your current surroundings and notice the sensations in your body. You are in safe hands.

Feeling Tones

An important concept to help you navigate your newfound connection to your body as an instrument of emotion is to understand feeling tones. I have referenced feeling tones throughout this book. Feeling tones present in your body as a temporary experience.

If we look at feeling tones through the lens of our conversation of the vagus nerve and chakras, feeling tones present by way of your thinking that activates your central nervous system and are experienced in your chakras. When you understand that feeling tones are temporary states, you can breathe and be mindful of them.

Here are the feeling tones that present in your body:

- Pleasant feeling tones
- Unpleasant feeling tones
- Neutral feeling tones

Meditation is a proven way to understand your feeling tones. Jon Kabbat-Zinn, the originator of Mindfulness Based Stress Reduction, says meditation is really a "non-doing" and that "it is the only human endeavor that emphasizes being where you already are."[53]

It's hard to experience the unpleasant feeling tones, but when you do, remember that you are okay. You will be safe when you allow yourself to do so. Experiencing with curiosity is the key. Feeling the "feels," being present, and observing without a dissociative quality is important to healing. This process sends signals throughout your system that you are capable of being present and aware. Over time, this becomes easier.

When I work with my clients in this way, I refer to this as "leaning in." Lean into the discomfort, and you will discover this part of

---

53. Kabbat-Zinn, *Full Catastrophe Living*, 55.

your body is carrying important information it needs you to understand. Your body is always and only in service of healing.

EXERCISE
Writing Prompt: Thank Your Body

In your journal, write a thank you note to your body. Thank it for what it has done for you this week. Be specific about the things it accomplished. Avoid being critical. Just thank your body.

If you care to, think about all your body has done for you over your lifetime. Has it gotten you out of some troubles through fight, flight, or freezing? After you do this, write the emotions that come up for you around this exercise, and notice where in your body you feel them.

Summary

Your body is the key to facilitating your spiritual experience as it engages with the world. It is not to be neglected as "unspiritual" since meaning and connection cannot be had without it. The body is key to registering both the pleasant and unpleasant experiences of your life. Being present to your body and being able to register if you are safe or unsafe is helped along with the metabolic responses of the vagus nerve. The root chakra is the grounding etheric force that helps you to stay firmly planted in the safety process as it registers energetic experiences.

If you have been unsafe in childhood, the vagus nerve and resulting chakric energy may misread safety cues because of old patterns. Understand that the body is the messenger for healing. Befriending the body because it is perceived as painful is the key to healing.

CHAPTER 5
EMOTIONS AND THE SACRAL CHAKRA

•————————•

Y ou need people. You don't need people to make you like yourself, but you need people to connect to in safe, affirming ways.

The sacral chakra governs your relationship to others. Located near the belly button, this energy is the source of attachment. It equips you to connect with others' emotional flow as you stay present to your own.[54] This is the region where your umbilical cord used to be—where you bonded with your first human being. In utero, you had all your essential needs met. How much you got your needs met after you were born—including how you were kept safe and loved by the person who birthed you—shaped the way you love others, including yourself, now.

This chakra both gives and receives powerful sources of psychological and physiological nourishment and care. It allows you to step fully into what you need.[55] It is associated with the color orange. Orange is not a primary color. It is a mixture of red and yellow. These are the colors of the chakras above and below it. The color orange is symbolic of the blending of body and mind, which generates the experience of emotion.

54. Saradananda, *Chakra Meditation*, 54.

55. Wauters, *Chakras and their Archetypes*, 51.

The sacral chakra is about how you partner in your community. Humans need the safety of connection—the village—to keep us alive and well. Within your community, you define what you need and negotiate to get those needs met. You also decide if you can meet another's needs.

This chakra reveals the patterns of your relationships. If you were respected, nurtured, and your realities were honored, you know where you physically and emotionally end and another begins. If your boundaries were honored growing up, then limit setting just "feels" right. If your caretakers were chaotic, abusive, or neglectful—if you were traumatized by those you loved—then most likely you don't feel safe enough to connect in your adult relationships. This reflects in your sacral chakra by restriction or too much intake or outflow. If you were dismissed, belittled, or experienced physical or psychological abuse from your caretakers, more than likely you struggle with identifying boundaries with others. You either take other peoples' emotions in and feel them as your own or you cannot clearly read the emotions of others or yourself. One is a flooding, the other a disconnect. Either way, this is felt in the sacral chakra.

As a child you engaged with people by observing how it was done. You developed social cues and values from watching, then trying out what you learned. This was first done in a family circle and then extended outwards as you grew into adulthood. This chakra represents your culturalization, which defines how you engage with the world and interpret others' messages. This chakra can be asked to do a lot of work as you grow and possibly change geographical locations and social customs throughout your life.

The Vagus Nerve and Your Sacral Chakra

The vagus nerve fibers that extend to the sacral chakra attach to the digestive organs, such as your stomach, large intestines, kidneys, and liver. These are visceral organs that encompass the area below the diaphragm. This region is called subdiaphragmatic. It is part of the more ancient threads of the nervous system: the dorsal vagal and the sympathetic nervous system. If you constantly worry, do you then "feel" fear through your back or stomach? Abdominal upset is an example of a visceral reaction.[56] Quite literally, emotions of unsafety are an inside out encounter. Just as with the part of the vagus nerve that aligns with your root chakra, the nerve fibers in this area that align with the sacral chakra are unmyelinated. This means the signals to and from this region of the body move slower because the nerves are not "coated" with a myelin sheath.[57] This creates less localized pain.

On the top of the kidneys sit two small glands called adrenals. They're not much larger than the upper portion of your thumb, but they're fierce defenders of you. Adrenals shoot cortisol into the system when you need to run from or fight off a threat. This part of the hypothalamic-pituitary-adrenal (HPA) axis is regulated through the vagus nerve. If your adrenals are constantly stimulated because you believe you're not safe, not loved, not wanted, not respected, not cared for, or not appreciated—all beliefs associated with the relational sacral chakra—cortisol streams into your system. Over time, your body will wear down and develop issues with fatigue.[58]

---

56. Sanossian and Haut, "Chronic Diarrhea Associated with Vagal Nerve Stimulation," 330.
57. Porges, Polyvagal Safety, 194.
58. Wilson, Adrenal Fatigue, 18.

When we *believe* we are safe or unsafe around others, this information is sent from the brain through the central nervous system. We can feel this in the sacral chakra. Safety relaxes this chakra. Lack of safety creates constriction in the sacral chakra.

When your body does not have to defend itself, you can extend yourself in a reliable and caring way to others.[59] How you see your world—and your relationship to people in it—is regulated through your physical systems and manifested outward into an energetic field with others.

Calming With Others

There is a very practical way to help ground yourself that includes loved ones, a beloved pet, or even a stuffed animal. This is called co-regulation. When you co-regulate, you're feeling the calming effects of another person. Specifically, your central nervous system and theirs are sending and receiving safety messages because you are both activating your ventral vagus nerve. Your relationships are key for the health of your central nervous system and body.

Co-regulation is done in therapy offices every day.[60] It's done in friendships, in families, with coworkers, and sometimes with strangers who extend a kindness. When we connect with those in safety, we get the same experience back. Your child's singing, the laughter of your best friend, and your partner's hug are signals that all is well.

Listening deeply and being heard is a huge form of co-regulation. Think back to a time when someone tended to you with no interruptions, nodding on occasion and affirming. Can you remember someone smiling, waving, and crossing the room to welcome you?

59. Ogden, Minton, and Pain, *Trauma and the Body*, 268.
60. Dana, *The Polyvagal Theory in Therapy*, 45–49.

What about when someone slowed their car to let you into traffic? What did you notice in your body?

The experience of co-regulation can occur when two people exchange knowing glances or sit quietly sipping coffee next to each other. When you are calm and your body is regulated, you feel this in your stomach, which is the center of your sacral chakra.

The physiological explanation for co-regulation utilizing the polyvagal theory goes back to ventral vagal (social) engagement. When we can read the upper portion of someone's face—their smile, how they make eye contact—our nueroception (the sense of our nervous system) tells us we are acknowledged, accepted, and loved. Our heart rate slows. Our muscles relax. Our blood pressure lowers.

The muscles in our face and throat soften when we feel safe, which allows us easy access to our voice. When we feel connected, we mirror that back to someone. The calming effects are uniting.

EXERCISE
Buddha Belly

Let's pull awareness to the sacral chakra. This exercise might go against the messages you have received about keeping your stomach tight and tucked in. When you regularly constrict the muscles around your waist, you're forcing the breath to the top part of your lungs only.

- To get a full breath, pull the air into your belly. See the air filling your stomach, and notice how this fills the bottom of your lungs. You will be engaging your whole torso in different ways. That requires softening the abdominal muscles (front stomach) so you can utilize the obliques (side muscles). See this as making space for all those organs we've been talking about. This exercise takes practice.

- Sit comfortably in your chair or on meditation cushions in your sacred space. Engage your spine without tensing. Just like in previous exercises, notice your bones and use them as a reference point for your posture.

- Now, draw a slow breath into your belly. Allow the abdominal muscles to relax. Imagine the stomach, liver, and intestines filling with air. Let the muscles create space inside of you, welcoming air into your body.

- Continue to just breathe. Nothing fancy. At times, notice how you feel sitting in the chair, then draw attention back to the stomach.

- How do your stomach and back feel as they get more oxygen?

- Focus your attention on the area around your belly button. Do you notice the energy of the sacral chakra? Sit with this for a while. What are you experiencing?

Equanimity: Highest Expression of the Emotional Dimension

Equanimity is the beat-by-beat awareness that keeps you whole-heartedly present and aware of what is occurring in your thoughts and body. The even, or "equal," attention to your process holds your emotional wheel steady. When you are able to do so, awareness is heightened and a healthy form of control (over you and no one else) becomes available. The mind always wants something more; equanimity creates a nearness that is balanced and subtle.

Being present to what your body is saying takes effort. Equanimity requires practice and intention. If you grew up around intensity and a lack of safety, you probably believed felt experience was too painful. You couldn't trust your emotions, and your mind learned to seek diversions from discomfort. More than likely, you worked hard to keep from being present.

Mindfully observing what is occurring between thoughts and body, which creates emotion, means being nonjudgmental and curious. By being equanimous, you are purposely curious and friendly with your thoughts and how they present in your body, which leads you to being deeply caring. Equanimity helps you establish a new relationship with yourself, which is how change starts. Being present is befriending yourself.

EXERCISE
Writing Prompt: The People around You

This prompt is designed to get you to understand your physiological responses in regard to your emotional connections with others. This can help you establish equanimity within yourself as you engage with people and the world differently.

- Who are the people I love?
- What other emotions do I feel for them?
- When I think about these people, how do I experience this in my sacral chakra?
- Are there other areas of my body where I feel strong emotion toward them?

Narrative: Lowest Expression
of the Emotional Dimension

Our past is a narrative. It's the meaning we made up once based on what happened in childhood. Perceiving a current situation based on the past means you're not seeing things for what they are now. You cannot be equanimous and in balance.

This does not mean the past wasn't part of a legitimate life story that potentially created pain for you. However, working from an old script keeps you locked in the place you least want to be in. It keeps us reacting in old ways and wondering why nothing changes.

Psychotherapist and Holocaust survivor Viktor Frankl discusses that healing from old narratives of oneself possesses a certain amount of tension and creates a "gap between what one is and what one should become."[61] How you choose to see or react to what is said or done by another is based on the meanings and beliefs you possess. You can read the old script and react with your old pattern. Another option might be to breathe, maybe literally stand back, and observe the situation by being curious. It's in that moment you can choose a different approach.

When you work from old emotional narratives, the energies around your chakras are tightened or loosened and hold memories of pain that are relayed to the central nervous system. Those energies show up in your whole system as the chakras are indicators of where you are psychologically.

Brittney's Story: Resetting Past Narratives

Brittney brought flowers to our first session. In a therapeutic relationship, gifts are frowned upon. They create a power dynamic

---

61. Frankl, *Man's Search for Meaning*, 105.

and can blur boundaries. I had to start the session by thanking her but letting her know I could not accept the flowers for this reason.

Her eyes grew large and appeared to fill with tears. She seemed confused and offended and suggested I wasn't "appreciative." Slumping her shoulders, she rested her hand on her stomach, where her sacral chakra is. When I asked why she was doing this, she called this her "pit of despair." Brittney was clearly locked in a pattern of offering things to people that could not reciprocate. This was leaving the energy in her sacral chakra too open and without limitations, which is why she was feeling that "pit of despair."

Brittney said she wanted to work on relationship issues. She was married for five years and had been divorced for three. She had no children. She told me that her biggest struggle was trying to maintain a consistent relationship with the men she was meeting online. She said she had no problem meeting guys, but they always left after the first month or so. The last man she dated had told her she was "suffocating" him.

"I think he was just emotionally unavailable," she said. "I'm a kind person. He was unappreciative."

"Hmmm," I said. "Did you not just suggest that of me?"

"Wow." She sat back and stared for a few seconds. "Yeah, I suppose I did."

As a massage therapist, Brittney spends her days healing others. She is body aware, practices yoga, understands the concepts of chakras, and can read the energies of others. She complained that at the end of each workday she felt exhausted, sometimes sick with headaches or other ailments including stomach issues. She stated she was proud that she could take away the pain from her clients even though sometimes she thinks she absorbed it into her own body.

In the first few sessions, she spent a considerable amount of time depicting the men she was interested in. She went dreamy when she described their physical qualities, what they said to her, and where they went on dates. When a man would not immediately text back, she grew despondent.

If she had a second date, Brittney grew wistful at the prospect of getting married again. We discussed what love addiction looked like, but she was not open to considering she was compulsively attempting to attach to people. Brittany always felt the men were the problem, that she just hadn't found one that "appreciated" her yet.

Brittney talked to her mother almost every day. Her mom called several times throughout the day from the retirement facility she was in. Each time she called, Brittney felt compelled to pick up the phone no matter how busy she was. Her father had died when she was in middle school, and her mother refused to talk about him or his death. Brittney said she was afraid to ask since this would upset her elderly mother.

"It was like one day he was sick and within a few months he was gone," she said. "Mom is still devastated all these years later and can't talk about it. She was so deeply in love with him."

"If your father was still here and hadn't left," I said, "what would you like to say to him?"

This question took her off guard. Her cheeks got red and flashes of anger crossed her face. Then, just as quickly, anger was gone, and she forced a smile. She looked up at me and said, "That I miss him."

"Even if he never left?"

"Oh." She was silent for a long time. "Then, I dunno."

That week, Brittney looked at her father's death certificate. He had died from cirrhosis of the liver. She came into our next session stunned. "Why wouldn't Mom tell me that? I didn't even know he drank."

"Can you talk to her about this?"

She shook her head. "I don't want to upset her."

Not upsetting the adults in her life, she was starting to see, was a common theme growing up. As the only child, Brittney had always been expected to act older than her years. If she did behave like a kid, she was chastised, or her parents withdrew from her.

"I think they just couldn't deal with any child energy in the house. They were older when they had me. My mother was anxious about noises. My father would always hide in his study when he was home. The house was so quiet." Brittney recalled drawing cards and making gifts for her parents in school. Not once did she remember getting an enthusiastic response. Over the years, the gifts and gestures from her became more frequent and elaborate. "I was determined to get affection from them."

"How do you think this plays out in your adult relationships now?"

"Hmmm. I do tend to be drawn to the guys who aren't as interested. The ones who want me don't seem to appeal to me."

Over time, Brittney was able to see how she had been attempting to connect to emotionally unavailable people by constantly giving and doing. When she found someone who was mildly interested in pursuing a relationship with her, she would overcompensate with gestures, gifts, scheduling the dates, and performing sexually before she was ready. This pushed them away and made them more unavailable, which made her more determined.

She was also able to see how she was doing this with her clients in her massage practice. "If they were scheduled for an hour but were in pain, I would always spend extra time with them."

She grimaced. "I think they started taking advantage of that, you know, pay for an hour and get an hour and twenty minutes."

Brittney and I broke down where she wanted to start setting boundaries and what that would look like. The easiest steps, she said, were with her clients. We decided she would stick to her schedules with them. No more extra twenty minutes. Soon she discovered that not only were clients booking and paying for longer sessions but she didn't feel so drained at the end of the day anymore.

It took her a while, but she eventually asked her mom not to call multiple times a day. They decided on once a day at a certain time. Brittney would not answer the phone if her mother called outside of their agreed upon time. It took her mother several weeks to abide by the plan—she tried using tears and complaining—but as Brittney's boundaries grew firmer, her mother honored the parameters. As it turned out, their conversations were more fruitful, and her mother also spent more time with friends and stopped turning to her daughter for a social outlet.

How Brittney approached dating was harder. With multiple Eye Movement Desensitization and Reprocessing (EMDR) sessions that targeted her old fears and pain about being neglected, she was able to process some of the compulsivity of wanting to fix things that didn't need fixing. We worked on emotions that allowed her to mourn her father. She started writing letters to him and was able to accurately identify what she felt. She grew comfortable with anger, which she was told she couldn't feel growing up. Being more fully engaged with how she was feeling allowed her to connect with people in ways that had appropriate limits.

Early on, I chose not to focus too much on movement or body work with Brittney. She was already engaged with energy work to the point of thinking that if she fixed this, her relationships would be better. It was actually the opposite. The energy in her sacral chakra was wide open because she enmeshed with people. In this case, her psychological work would heal her etheric energy. A healthy pattern of connection through knowing her own limits alleviated her "pit of despair." Setting emotional, psychological, and physical limits based on her family patterns was what put a natural reset to this etheric energy for her.

Relationships as a Reflection of Self

Relationships are not just necessary for your body to survive but for your authentic Self to thrive. You can learn so much about who you are as you engage with people. You possess complex traits as a human being, and these reflect back at you through dynamics with others.[62] Your interpersonal connections offer tremendous opportunities to understand yourself. Your vagus nerve and etheric energy are in heightened awareness around others as you continually search for safety from others through understanding, kindness, and acceptance.

This is reflected in the people you choose to be around. (Remember my light bulb theory from chapter 1?) Think for a moment about those you are most drawn to. What qualities do you admire in them? Are they funny and lighthearted? Are they devoted? Do they possess a sense of social justice and empathy? Do they care for their family? Are they heavy drinkers? Do they obsess about the social status and money of others for their own self gain? Are they kind or cruel? Angry? Gossipy and judgmental? Inconsistent? What is the overarching theme in your relationships with the people in your life? The personality traits you admire or are drawn to in others are the traits you possess and admire

---

62. McConnell, *Somatic Internal Family Systems Therapy*, 128.

in yourself. This is also true about the characteristics you want to disown or dislike in yourself. Fixations on another's flaws are only deflections of aspects of you. When you decline to acknowledge them, you don't have to take responsibility for them. For example, if you can allow yourself to be sidetracked by the ineptitude of another, you delay the journey that takes you deeper into your own feeling of unworthiness.

A good thought to remember: if you point a finger at others, you are really pointing it back at yourself.

Emotional Boundaries

Loving acceptance of who you are leads to connecting with your Soul Self. This creates ventral vagal safety in your vagus nerve. Engaging kindly with yourself tells your system you are secure. When you know what you feel, how you think, and what you care about, you can identify your needs. You take yourself out of sympathetic engagement because you no longer feel uncertain. This is what it takes to develop emotional boundaries because the more securely placed within yourself you are, the easier it is to not let harmful, confusing energies in.

A boundary protects. What it protects are the things you value. When you think of a boundary, do you see it as securing only your physical belongings, such as property or your body? What do emotional boundaries look like to you?

Qualities such as your thoughts, feelings, visualizations, creative ideas, fantasies, hopes, and spiritual or political beliefs are some of the things that make up your inner world. When you understand your values, it becomes easy to want to safeguard them. You get to decide what you want to share and with whom.

Understanding what makes up your emotional inner world and setting limits with others who might violate it brings peace.

How can you tell when someone is attempting to break down your emotional boundaries? It's easy to know if someone disrespects or violates a physical boundary. You can see it. Emotional boundary violations are invisible. You can't see them, but you can feel them. A violation of an emotional boundary can range from an unintended misstep that hurt someone's feelings to full-on emotional, psychological, and mental abuse. Because emotional boundaries are not tangible, people can get confused about where their psychological self ends and someone else's begins.

Has someone denied your reality of a situation? Have you been mocked for experiencing a situation differently than someone else? When a person tells you what to feel or says your feelings are not accurate, how does that show up in your body? Where do you feel these experiences in your body?

Here's an even harder question to answer. Have you ever violated another's emotional boundaries? Have you told others how they should or shouldn't feel? Children are easily manipulated in this way, and it's up to us adults to be careful of this.

More examples of emotional boundary violations are:

- Calling people names
- Ignoring someone
- Eye rolling
- Telling someone they're wrong about their opinion
- Denying someone the right to express themselves
- Laughing at a person
- Gossiping
- Character assassinating someone

When someone is attempting to push those boundaries, you have a very clear indicator of how that feels. It's a physical sense. Slow down and check in with your body. Does the sensation of being hurt, invaded, pushed around, exhausted, angry, annoyed, agitated, impatient, or creeped out by someone's actions or words come up for you? The energy in your sacral chakra should give you a strong clue. Perhaps other chakras will feel that violation as well. Being emotionally violated also shows up through the central nervous system as your system is sending signals that something is wrong.

When you know what your emotional priorities are, you are less inclined to be manipulated. It's when you don't have a grounded sense of yourself that you can easily be pushed out of your center because you don't feel safe. Lines in relationships become blurred. Uncertainty and confusion create chaos and that keeps you in sympathetic engagement from your vagus nerve. That looks like anxiety and fear.

Trust what your body is telling you about potential emotional violations. Your body does not lie about how you are feeling.

EXERCISE
Defining Emotional Boundaries Using a Value Circle

Below is an exercise I love to do with my clients. I call it a "Value Circle." You do this for your physical values as well as your emotional values. Separating the two helps you understand the difference between physical, or "outer," boundaries and emotional, or "inner," boundaries. The clearer you are about what is important to you, the easier it will be to stop others from crossing that invisible line.

You already possess inner values. You have always had them. However, just like your talents, you're so close to your inner values you probably don't know what they are. Sometimes you have to dig deep just to touch the things that are right beside you.

Values are what you already employ. You engage in your world every day through your value system. A good way to decipher what your values are is by asking how you connect with others in the world. Look at the people you choose to spend time with and ask yourself what you have in common. You will see how they mirror your values back at you.

Another way to look at values is by asking what qualities you are drawn to in others. You might feel that you want those qualities but don't possess them. However, if you value them, put them in the circle. These might be emerging within you. Doing this exercise sets intention. Knowing what you value helps you define what you are safeguarding.

So, let's explore what you value emotionally. I always recommend to my clients to do this in a journal and to revisit this value circle over time. You can also put this on your refrigerator and look at it everyday to reinforce your values.

- Draw a larger circle that expands to the edges of the paper.
- Within that circle, draw another circle, making enough space to write in between the edges of both circles.
- The large circle and the space up to the line of the smaller circle will be the area where you write what you value physically. What are those things? They can be as simple as your house or car. Keep thinking of all that you value that is tangible.

- When you have written down as many physical values as you can think of, go to the inner circle. Write down as many values that make up your inner world that you can think of. Be specific. For instance, don't just write *spirituality* or *creative expression*. Instead, write what kind of spirituality is important to you or what kind of creative expression you value (e.g., writing, painting in acrylics, playing guitar, etc.).
- You may not have a lot in your inner circle yet. You may have a ton. Keep this page open throughout the week. Return to it as you continue to ask yourself what you value.

What I'm trying to do with this exercise is help you increase your awareness of what's significant.

As a caveat, if you're inclined to people please and hear the word *should* as you write, then investigate what is true for you versus what someone told you. Are you writing what you think you should value because you've been told to value it? Ironically, telling someone what they value is a huge violation of an emotional boundary.

Evolution is part of inner growth. Our values shift over time. Values that are more important now may not have been ten years ago. For that reason, this exercise is always fun to return to over the years.

Holding the Wheel Firmly

Now that you know what you value, you can settle more deeply into who you already are. This will reflect outward into the work you do, the choices you make, and the people you choose to be around. You may find self-care is easier. You might discover being with yourself is more enjoyable. You might lean into talents you didn't want to develop before.

It takes work to recognize when an emotional line has been crossed because it takes work to know what our emotional lines are. Remember, this is *your* reality. It may not be the other person's. That other person may be forceful when you express how you feel. Or perhaps their response is more covert but still denying. When you're attuned to what you feel, people who want to convince you otherwise will be less inclined to do so because they will feel your limit.

Knowing an emotional line has been crossed—and being able to express that—ensures your individuality, which ensures your inner safety. No one can truly break through your emotional boundaries unless you let them. People can affect how you feel, but they cannot determine what you choose to do with those feelings. They cannot determine the course of your actions unless you allow it to happen.

Some boundaries may simply require that you step out of the role of overfunctioning for others. You may find that handing over responsibilities that you had taken on, which weren't even yours in the first place, is all that you need to do.

The more emotional attachment and history we have with a person, the murkier this new way of communicating can be. Even when both people are attempting to break out of old patterns, this process is difficult. While boundaries need to be firm, they also need to be flexible. Different boundaries are required for different situations.

The Rule of Threes

I like to tell my clients that there seems to be three kinds of people who will mess with your newly established emotional boundaries.

The first is what I call *the healthy person*. They may have pushed your boundaries because you have never fully set a limit before.

They may not be aware that they are crossing emotional lines with you. This person, once they understand where your limit is, respects the new boundary. You may even find that person feels some relief since they are now able to know what you want and need. They can respond accordingly.

I call the second person in this "rule of threes" *the toddler*. This person may repeatedly come back to test these new limits, acting like a two-year-old who wants to make sure you really mean what you say. They want to see if you're serious about sticking their finger in that electrical socket. They may be initially uncomfortable with this new you since your change is forcing them to change. The test for these people is if they stay or leave once you are consistent with your new limit. If they leave, then they weren't with you for the right reasons.

The third and worst kind of person in this "rule of threes" is *the toxic person*. They will not listen to this new boundary and may do whatever it takes to manipulate or intimidate you out of setting limits with them. Your new perimeters are not convenient to them. They see any attempt at setting limits as a personal rejection. If they can't push that new boundary back down while directly engaging with you, they may use covert tactics. Covert tactics look like gossiping to others about you or assassinating your character. Character assassination employs others to continue the gossip about you. If they can't wear you down directly, they will use others to achieve their means. The toxic person has no interest in honoring your well-being. This person is dangerous and detrimental to your sanctity. You will have to leave this relationship.

EXERCISE
Emotional Boundary Script

Sometimes, when boundaries need to be set with others, you need a script to effectively communicate your needs. The following exercise is another activity I do with my clients and is a compilation of techniques I have learned over the years. This script gives you a clear picture of what you value internally because you must first be clear within yourself about what you need. I suggest doing this exercise in your journal. Think of someone you would like to ask something of as a way to practice.

Here's the format:

Clearly define **the issue** you're struggling with.

Stay specific: *When you told me last night that we're going to the movies Friday night no matter what.*

Not: *When we go out on Friday night.*

Clearly define **your thought** about this. Don't use blaming tactics.

Again, be specific: *What I thought was, 'you don't care about what I want to do Friday night.'*

Not: *You were being stupid and ignorant!*

Clearly define **your feelings** about this. Make sure you don't pull in more thoughts.

Stay specific to feelings that present in your body: *I felt ignored, bullied, angry, and sad.*

Not: *You always make me upset about this, and I feel that you don't care about me!*

Clearly define **your future expectation** about this:

In the future, I need you to ask me what I want to do on our date night.

Not: *You need to be more considerate!*

Remember, when you know what you value and when you can decipher your emotions, you can ask for what you need. The sacral chakra is the energetic opening that can at once connect to others but signal what is real in you. Paying attention to how your body feels through your chakras and how your central nervous system is responding plays a strong role in this.

Summary

For us to feel safe, we need to understand boundaries are not just physical. Emotional boundaries play an important part in healthy relationships. If you suffered childhood trauma of any kind, emotional boundaries were not honored. Therefore, it might be hard for you to understand what your emotional limits are—or that you have them—as you engage with others. Becoming aware of your physical cues through your sacral chakra and noticing signals of safety through the vagus nerve can help you identify emotional boundary violations.

Reclaiming emotional wholeness also involves developing the skill set to be present to your internal values. Identifying when others are not honoring your limits and developing ways to maintain those limits is vital. Challenging old narratives takes work and requires support. Equanimity is the result of being present to your etheric and physical systems.

CHAPTER 6
MIND AND THE
SOLAR PLEXUS CHAKRA

———•———

The solar plexus chakra is your personality power center. It's the shimmering light that charges you. It's your crusading force. This energy reflects who you are in the world and how you are in relation to others. The solar plexus is the lower case "self" that forms your identity with the outside world, free will in an incarnate body, and desire to achieve.

Once your basic needs are formed in infancy (root chakra) and your connection to caretakers and others is established (sacral chakra), you begin to define your place among your peers with the energy of the solar plexus chakra.

This chakra is located in the crux of the rib cage between and below the lungs. Yellow is its color. It shines bright like the sun and sometimes, like the sun, it burns. It's the last of the essential chakras that make up your survival instincts. It's also associated with your individuation. So, too, is your mind.

Mind, in this case, is the way in which you perceive your world—not the function of the brain.[63] Knowing your mind is how you possess agency over your life. Understanding that you perceive

---

63. Siegel, *The Developing Mind*, 214.

your own reality can give you space between your thoughts and your body.

True power lies in knowing that controlling things outside of you with distractions is a deception of self.[64] Taking responsibility for your choices and thought patterns and honoring when they are misleading you is key to a balanced connection to this energy source. When your mind refuses to see situations for what they are, you seek semblance through illusions. This is magical thinking. Magical thinking is wanting things to be what you want despite evidence to the contrary. You then work hard to maintain illusions. You hold on to old narratives that comfort you but do you little good. This creates confusing signals of safety in your system because you can't accurately assess a situation. There's no opportunity for flexibility of thought when you work through magical thinking because you are needing to be right just to keep the illusions going.

Through this perspective, you're in a power-over, power-under way of engaging with people.[65] The lens you see life through becomes about who is right. Seeking power-over is powerlessness. Your chakras, and energy in general, become distorted and churn in dysregulated ways. The sunshine, which normally charges you, burns you. Vitality becomes stasis. When this happens, aspects of intimacy, communication, emotions, and appetite are overcharged in the body, and you struggle to get the true connection your Soul Self craves. This can either overload or shut down the energy center of your solar plexus.

Utilizing mind for a greater good, including what is best within yourself, helps to keep your frequency burning more evenly. Compassion is the key. Applying softer thoughts for yourself and others slows thing down and balances things out. When you are able to

---

64. Kabbat-Zinn, *Full Catastrophe Living*, 326.
65. Evans, *Controlling People*, 10.

recognize your thinking and be more curious as to the root of it, you can free up space in both your head and your body for acceptance.[66]

The Solar Plexus Chakra and the Vagus Nerve

Applying knowledge of your vagus nerve and thinking patterns provides you the opportunity to manage the energy in this chakra. The vagus nerve connects the solar plexus through the upper portion of the digestive system along with the kidneys and adrenals.[67] This is the endocrine system we discussed in previous chapters.

The endocrine system controls when and how your body reacts to stress. When you overthink, worry, blame, rage, or need to be right—which are all illusions of the mind—you stimulate the fight, flight, and sometimes freeze responses. The emotional brain ignites, sending alarms to the system that it's in danger. You feel that burning through the solar plexus. This shows up through cortisol release in your body that it doesn't need and with intestinal issues that may appear to be medical but are exclusively emotional and neurophysiological reactions to the stressors of your thoughts.

Signals of danger run down the unmyelinated nerve fibers, and your body perceives its basic needs are threatened. Not only is the solar plexus chakra then overactivated but the other essential chakras of the root and sacral are as well. You might buckle over and press your arms and hands to your stomach in a protective gesture because the area around your solar plexus burns. You might want to run or walk it out given the system is activated for a lack of safety and it wants to move.

---

66. Brach, *Radical Compassion*, 112.
67. Porges and Dana, *Clinical Applications of the Polyvagal Theory*, 59.

Another aspect of mind, which we will discuss in more detail in later chapters, has to do with how your brain is registering information through synaptic changes. You store memories through a very complicated system that incorporates all three levels of the brain. Understanding that your brain holds information through neurotransmitters that run along a system of pathways, called neuropathways, is important as these pathways strengthen over time. When events repeat themselves, especially when the brain is developing, and thoughts and beliefs solidify as truths, behaviors and responses are amplified.

In extremely simple terms, the more you repeat a thought, the deeper that neuropathway becomes ingrained in your system. These thoughts are constantly signaling the central nervous system to respond. When that pattern is repeatedly fired, the information encodes, and the network remembers these patterns as truth.

No pill, no amount of binging, no restriction of food, alcohol, or any substance that attempts to soothe this discomfort will heal you long term. Knowing how your system got activated in the first place—in this case, by your thought patterns and the meaning made by them—and healing early childhood wounds that form your current reality, will. Management of your mind—knowing what you think versus feel—helps you trust this human paradox, which can alleviate anxiety.

Difference Between Anxiety and Emotion

What I just described in the previous section is an example of anxiety. Anxiety is a physiological response to your state of mind. It's brought on by conflicting and worrying thoughts that create reactions in your central nervous system. Anxiety is not emotion.

Emotions are the softer, deeper, and kinder energies that are present in your body at various times and flow from the wiser guidance of your Soul Self.[68] Emotions can be embraced. They have poignancy and subtlety. Even what is perceived as a difficult emotion, such as sadness, anger, or fear, can be tender in your system. Companioning your emotions becomes easy and not threatening when we can understand how they appear and feel in your system.

Thoughts, however, are rapid and tricky. They seek outcome, not presence. It's easy to get tripped up by thoughts that demand immediate results. Thoughts are inconsistent, sometimes harsh. They can appear in an instant and are gone before you can identify what happened.

Recent studies have shown we have thousands of thoughts a day.[69] They are the driving sensors in your vehicle and are on constant alert based on your past experiences. Many don't apply to your current circumstances but don't know that.

New clients are shocked to hear there is a difference between anxiety and emotion. So many of us—probably most of us—initially spend our lives unable to discern between the two. Children on high alert experience the emotions of sadness, anger, or loneliness with a blend of anxiety that comes from a lack of physical or emotional safety. It's no wonder that, as an adult, you find ways to disconnect from your body. Your mind has perceived that feeling emotion is the same as experiencing an overcharged threat in your central nervous system.

Identities of self are formed through your thoughts and how you negotiate your place in the world. These characteristics of

68. McConnell, *Somatic Internal Family Systems Therapy*, 15–16.
69. Tseng and Poppenk, "Brain Meta-State Transitions Demarcate Thoughts Across Task Contexts Exposing the Mental Noise of Trait Neuroticism."

who you are may have conflicting ideas about how to go about things. It's these clashing beliefs that can stimulate your sympathetic nervous system. While aspects of you are of your mind, you most certainly feel their outcome all over your body. I am trained in Internal Family Systems (IFS) therapy. It's an approach to therapy that honors that we have multiplicity in our identity. Just like members in a family, your thoughts and beliefs may clash about how to approach an issue. Do you sometimes feel you have multiple thoughts, or what I call a "family food fight at the table" happening?

EXERCISE
How Many Thoughts?

This is an exercise I use with my clients to help them sort through the various—sometimes conflicting—aspects in their mind. Visualizing your conflicting thoughts as people may help you sort through the anxiety you may be experiencing about an issue.

- As always, find a comfortable place for you to sit and get your journal. Remind yourself that you are in a safe, comfortable space. Take a few breaths and center yourself.
- Think of a problem you are trying to work through. Write the problem out on paper so you can be clear in your mind about what the problem is. As you write, notice how your body feels.
- Once you have written the problem out, notice each conflicting thought you have around that problem and write them down. Flesh out all varying opinions. You may have a few on paper, or you may have many.

- See each of those conflicting thoughts as people or archetypes (they could also be a texture, form, or color) that are presenting their own opinion of the situation.
- As you let them speak, give them an opportunity to stand behind or beside you. As if these were real family members, let them each take a turn. Tell them to wait their turn until the other one finishes. What do you see?
- As you listen to them talk, notice how your body feels. Is there anxiety? If so, where? Breathe and remind yourself that you are safe. What they have to say is their own perspective. They are neither right nor wrong, just simply looking at an issue in their own way.
- After they have shared their views, thank them for the work they are doing. Whether or not other parts agree with them, just honor them. Let them know they were heard.
- Now, just notice your body. Is it calmer?
- These parts of your mind are the identities you utilize to help you manage your world. Thank them for their good intentions.

Discernment: The Higher Expression of Mind

When you discern, you're making decisions based on inner awareness and being attuned to your needs. You're present. You're intentional in your fairness. Discerning allows you to make intelligent, healthy choices that reflect your inner awareness. It just feels right since the answer to the question is coming from a deeper place within you. Discernment means you have healthy emotional boundaries because you know what you value. Knowing yourself is your power source.

To discern takes equanimity. Equanimity is striving for balance and truthfulness within yourself that reflects outward to others. This takes awareness of what you're thinking and feeling and how you communicate this. Discernment not only reflects an awareness of what is happening for you but to others. When you understand yours can be a separate experience, you can stay true to your inner self but open to the ideas and realities of others.

If you can pause and reflect, check in with your body, you're working from a place of gentle strength. I like to think of discernment as a muscle that needs to be flexed over and over for it to be used well. Maintaining an awareness of your own system's responses can help you gain a deeper awareness of your state of mind. You can also take measure of how your energy system affects those around you.

In Japan, there is the phrase *kuuki wo yomu*. Loosely translated, it means "reading the air." It is a nonverbal approach to being responsive to the collective mood of the people in the room, or the effect you're having on another and how their system is affecting yours. Matching with another's body language is a way to understand and join with a person. Kuuki wo yomu forces you to be present.

Judgment: The Lower Expression of Mind

Easy is the mind that will not judge, for therein lies a peace-filled life. There are no boundaries with judgment. Judgment is an energetic attempt to violate the private domain and integrity of others. When you judge, you're condemning and attempting to damage relationships and reputations. Judging distances you from people and experiences. It's an effort to control by dismissing.

The process of judging has components of boredom to it because judgment can fill the time in your head. When you're bored and don't like what is occurring within yourself, you seek diversions. It's a psychological prop to hide behind. It's a way to avoid uncomfortable, disowned aspects of yourself. Judging is an attempt to dump your hurts onto another person. When you openly (and inwardly) spend time judging others, you're absorbing their karma into your own psyche.

When you're truthful with yourself, you're able to look at how the habit of judging keeps your illusions functioning. Those illusions are hard to crack. They protect precious things like low self-esteem, fears, sadness, anger, longing for acceptance, broken attachments, or fear of abandonment. When you don't know another way of managing yourself, you hold dear to defenses of the mind.

EXERCISE
Looking into the Mirror

This exercise requires you to be deeply honest with yourself. Sometimes we must sit in the discomfort of our disowned coping mechanisms to face our hurts and open our hearts.

- Reflect on a time you talked negatively about someone. What did you say?
- Notice, as you reflect, if you get defensive about why you did this.
- Is your mind seeking a narrative that justifies talking about them? Just notice.

- Breathe as you stay aware of the moment you talked about them.
- Slow your mind down and take another deep breath.
- Now ask yourself, "What is the quality in them that I don't like about myself?"
- Take a deeper breath. This is the hard part.
- Be aware of what is happening in your body as you do this.

Reflecting on the aspect of someone you deeply dislike and being truthful about how this reflects your own disowned parts is powerful. It won't destroy you. It allows you deep insight. It takes bravery and maturity to reflect this deeply.

Sometimes answering this question requires the help of a professional. Those qualities we dislike in ourselves are deeply buried beneath decades of coping mechanisms we believe we need. Vilifying another does not bring us closer to ourselves. It profoundly disconnects us.

Taryn's Story: When Anxiety Controls the Family

Taryn identifies as nonbinary. They struggled to make this known outside of the LGBTQ community since the one time they shared this with their parents, their mother and father threatened to send them to conversion camp.

For the first month Taryn and I started working together, they were so anxious, it was hard for them to stay seated. Taryn struggled with communicating their story and could not focus on one issue for long.

Taryn's parents expected certain things from their child's academic performance. However, their parents didn't want Taryn to leave their small town to go to a better college. Taryn eventually left and was going to college in the city when they came to me. Every other weekend, Taryn made the long drive home because they feared for their parent's well-being. Taryn's parents also asked that they all stay on a family GPS system since they were afraid something would happen to Taryn.

Over time, Taryn's girlfriend, Sasha, started asking for similar demands. Sasha would ask Taryn for regular check-ins. Exhausted and overwhelmed by the constant demands from people they cared about, Taryn started shutting down. Taryn complained of adrenal fatigue and said their solar plexus was always churning. They dissociated and struggled being present in class. They would sleep for hours at a time during the day. Taryn reported not feeling in their body most days.

"How do you feel about having to constantly let people know where you are?" I asked.

"Like a child. I just can't do this anymore."

"You don't have to be responsible for managing other people's anxiety," I said.

Understanding flashed over Taryn's face. "Oh, wow, is this what I'm doing?"

"Sometimes anxious people think if they can control things outside of themselves, including their kids," I gestured to Taryn, "they expect the anxiety will go away."

They nodded. "I can totally see this!"

"And do you feel you control your anxiety by keeping them happy and doing what they want you do to?"

"Holy cow, yes!"

We came up with a plan that included firm boundaries, knowing that both parents would attempt to push back for a while. We discussed how giving them space to work through their own "stuff" and not be their parents' constant diversion would naturally reset everyone's energy.

It took some time and some regular practice on Taryn's part, but boundaries were followed through with. Taryn's parents pulled on them less and less. Sasha respected Taryn's privacy, too, as she could see what her demands were doing to the relationship and Taryn. Soon, Taryn was able to have enough physical and emotional space that allowed them to hear their own needs.

EXERCISE
Writing Prompt: Fleshing Out Feelings

Let's discern how your mind interprets feelings. The following is a list of three basic feelings: anger, happiness, and sadness. We know there are degrees of these feelings.

- In your journal, make a column header for these three feelings.
  - Anger
  - Happiness
  - Sadness
- Beneath each feeling, list the qualities you can identify with the feeling. For instance, a degree of anger can be annoyance. A degree of happiness can be gleeful. A degree of sadness can be solemness.
- List as many qualities as you can on your own first. Then, if you need to, look at the examples that follow.

Examples of the Qualities of the Basic Emotions
The following is an extensive list of the different qualities of the
three basic emotions.

- Disgust
- Contempt
- Revulsion
- Envy
- Jealousy
- Exasperation
- Frustration
- Irritation
- Aggravation
- Agitation
- Annoyance
- Grouchiness
- Grumpiness
- Rage
- Bitterness
- Dislike
- Ferocity
- Fury
- Hate
- Hostility
- Loathing
- Outrage
- Resentment
- Scorn
- Spite
- Vengefulness
- Wrath
- Torment
- Fear
- Alarm
- Fright
- Horror
- Hysteria
- Mortification
- Panic
- Shock
- Terror
- Apprehension
- Distress
- Dread
- Nervousness
- Tenseness
- Uneasiness
- Worry
- Joy
- Cheerfulness
- Amusement
- Bliss
- Delight
- Ecstasy
- Elation
- Enjoyment
- Euphoria
- Gladness

- Glee
- Jolliness
- Joviality
- Joy
- Jubilation
- Satisfaction
- Contentment
- Optimism
- Eagerness
- Hope
- Relief
- Enthusiasm
- Excitement
- Exhilaration
- Zeal
- Adoration
- Affection
- Compassion
- Fondness
- Love
- Sentimentality
- Tenderness
- Disappointment
- Dismay
- Displeasure

- Defeat
- Dejection
- Rejection
- Embarrassment
- Homesickness
- Hopelessness
- Loneliness
- Humiliation
- Insecurity
- Isolation
- Insult
- Neglect
- Despair
- Gloom
- Misery
- Sorrow
- Woe
- Shame
- Guilt
- Regret
- Remorse
- Hurt
- Suffering
- Anguish

This exercise is a good opportunity to reflect on what thoughts, memories, or associations you might have that bring up these emotions. Does anything about the various qualities of these emotions surprise you?

Metacognitions

Thinking is a habit. Most of what is going through your mind is ground you've already covered, perhaps for years. When you can identify your thinking patterns, you can shift them. You can distinguish how your mind creates emotions and develop a more acute awareness that will facilitate different outcomes.

A metacognition is a way of "thinking about what you're thinking."[70] It is an advanced form of processing your inner world. You are able to stand back and observe yourself in the process of your thoughts and establish how they are affecting you physiologically. This raising of consciousness influences the way you interact with your world and increases adaptability. You can then see that you might have various outcomes in a situation and can take responsibility for the choices you make. Metacognitively working through things requires you to slow down enough to notice what is occurring in your mind. You can observe the various forms your thinking takes, including objective or subjective patterns.

Objectivity is based in facts, such as numbers and measurements. It can generally be applied to linear thinking as it requires measurement and outcome. Scientific thinking is based in objectivity. Utilizing objective thinking means you are striving to be impartial. Having an objective is different. This is usually the result of thinking and means you are focused on an end goal. It doesn't necessarily mean you are thinking objectively.

Subjective realities are what we think is happening. We utilize subjectivity when we make decisions based on personal experience, emotions, tastes, or desired outcomes. Subjective thinking boils down to personal tastes, or perhaps what we want from a

---

70. Shannon and Frischherz, *Metathinking*, 35.

situation. It can be formed based on family narratives and child-hood experiences.

Have you and a sibling ever shared stories from your past? Are you surprised they have a different version of the story than you? Theirs is not wrong. It's how they made meaning of that shared experience. Two people. Two different interpretations.

Metacognition is a way to affect the outcome in your central nervous system and chakras. When you can see your pattern of thinking and are aware of the cause and effect of a thought on your body, you can develop enough flexibility of mind to work toward ventral vagal soothing if need be. How your narrative creates safety or lack of safety for the system is part of "thinking about what you're thinking." As you go about your day, just notice your thoughts. Check in with your heart rate, your stomach, your breathing, and the energy of your chakras. Your thoughts do not own you. You own your thoughts.

EXERCISE
The Johari Window

The Johari Window is a great exercise for self-exploration.[71] It can help you understand your mind and how you see your world. The four windowpanes represent aspects of yourself that you may or may not be aware of. Start with the upper left corner, then move to the lower left. The third window to work through is the upper right. The fourth window, the lower right, is the hardest window to compose and will take time.

---

71. Luft and Ingham, "The Johari Window."

- The first pane, perhaps the easiest to work with, represents qualities of yourself that you and others know about you.

- The second window asks you to explore aspects of yourself that others do not know about you. This is where it's helpful to understand the difference between privacy and shame. Privacy has boundaries around it. These are things you share only with those you trust. Secrets carry shame. These are the parts you hide from others because you are embarrassed. As you fill this out and see some of these aspects are secretive, I want to encourage you not to shame yourself further. Know that when worked through, these secrets can become private and not shame filled.

- The top right pane might require you to ask friends and family about what they know about you that you don't know about yourself. This is a wonderful way to emotionally explore and stretch.

- The bottom right window is the one that takes the most reflection. What are facets of you that are not known to others and that you are not aware of yet? One of the pathways into this corner is to notice how you think. What are the patterns? This requires some reflection and time. Meditation can deepen this connection to yourself.

These unknown aspects don't have to be shameful or hurtful. They could be aspirations that are deeply buried. An example from my own life is how I decided I wanted to change careers and become a counselor. I was personally driven by spiritual and psychological growth and was intrigued by the counseling profession. The seeds had always been there. I had never considered being one until life changes pushed me deeper into myself. I had to ask, "What drives me, and what else do I want to do with my life?" Sometimes it takes events outside of us to understand the qualities inside of us.

The Johari Window

	Known to Self	Not Known to Self
Known to Others	Open/Arena	Blind Spot
Not Known to Others	Hidden/Façade	Unknown

Figure 3: The Johari Window

How to Cultivate Mind to Serve a Higher Purpose

If you're in constant stress because of the way you think, more than likely you're not being very kind to you or those around you. The greatest challenge is to recognize and dispute beliefs that stimulate your anxiety and create destructive behaviors. The following is a list of some of these thought patterns. Do you recognize yourself in these? This list of cognitive distortions is loosely derived from cognitive behavioral theory but has been expounded upon through other sources through the years.[72]

---

72. "Resources for Professionals and Students."

- **All or nothing:** "It's either this way or nothing." This leads to chaotic or rigid boundaries.
- **Catastrophizing:** "If this doesn't happen, life is over." This is constant overstimulation of the sympathetic nervous system.
- **Logical:** "You are not making sense." This keeps from feeling emotions.
- **Mind reading:** "I know what you're thinking." This enables passive-aggressive behaviors.
- **Labeling:** "You know how they are." This leads to racist, misogynist, or misanthropic aggression.
- **Minimizing:** "It's not that bad." This creates disconnection of emotions or denying yours or others' realities.
- **Discounting the positive:** "This good thing was a fluke." This instills depression.
- **Shoulds:** "You should be doing something and not relaxing." This is an inability to be present.
- **Personalizing:** "The people at this party don't like me." This justifies victimhood.

EXERCISE
Solar Plexus Meditation

A mindful approach to observing how you think naturally instills a calmer mindset and body. Tara Brach, Buddhist monk and author, suggests utilizing the skill of identifying your thoughts. For instance, as judgments arise, name them, "Judging, judging, judging."[73] This helps you separate from the illusion that your thoughts are the only truth. When you can do this, the

---

73. Brach, *Radical Compassion*, 25.

region around your solar plexus and your sympathetic nervous system settle. I would also suggest that, if you feel anxiety arise, you offer the thought "I am safe" and notice how it affects your experience.

- Sit quietly in a chair or pillow of your choice. Keep your spine straight but not tense.
- Set one hand on your solar plexus and connect to the vitality in this part of your body.
- Does the energy change when you set your palm on this chakra?
- Rest your other hand on your thigh to balance yourself and close your eyes.
- Focus on the quality of your breath without changing how you are breathing.
- Notice your breaths. Where do they flow into your body? Are they cool? Warm?
- As thoughts arise, be curious without following them to conclusion.
- Say to yourself, "There's a thought." Don't judge the thought. Let them float by, and go back to focusing on your breath. Use your breath as the grounding point.
- Notice how the breath is affecting this energy center in your body.
- Remind yourself that you are safe. Notice how this affects the solar plexus.
- Does knowing you are safe change the quality of the energy in your chakra?

Mental Boundaries

In the last chapter, we discussed setting emotional boundaries by understanding what you value. Mental boundaries are equally as important. How you think, just as much as how you feel, grounds you into place. It creates a wholeness in you and defines you as an autonomous individual.

Clarity of thought is a boundary. When you are sure about what you are thinking, you can be clear with others. It doesn't leave anyone confused.

One of the ways people attempt to violate another's mental boundaries and steal psychic energy is by denying the reality of that person. Gaslighting is a pop-psych term that describes this behavior.[74] Gaslighting is a form of manipulation. Its intent is to get someone to doubt their beliefs, memories, or perceptions. There is a power-over dynamic that occurs in gaslighting.

An uncertain person will install all sorts of other tactics in an effort to keep someone off center about their thoughts. They may not understand they are doing it, as the idea of boundaries around thoughts is rarely ever discussed when approaching healthy ways of being.

Know your mind. Listen to your "gut." When you do this, you establish a firm identity. Utilize the energy of your body. Those essential chakras will not lead you astray. They will help you discern your unique truth. The energy of your chakras that results from the messaging in your central nervous system is the energy of your Soul. If there is one thing in your life that will not lead you astray, it is your Soul.

---

74. "Gaslighting," *Psychology Today*.

EXERCISE
Writing Prompt: Reality Is Relative with Relatives

We've been talking a lot about the subjectivity of your thoughts. Identifying what they are and gauging them with the outer world assists you in determining your reality. The act of journaling on its own reveals that.

When we are with family, sometimes our reality does not match up with family members' realities. At times this is frustrating, at times it's painful. Let's explore your perceptions of your place in your family or friend system with these writing prompts.

- What are ways you remember having a reality that didn't match up with someone else's, like a parent or sibling?
- What did they say happened (or didn't)?
- How did this situation affect you? How did your family member or friend say it affected them?
- Did you come to an understanding that you both share different views of the situation?
- How did you come to that agreement?

Remember that just because you share a different reality than another person, they are not necessarily wrong. Providing space for what they think is practicing boundaries from the "outside." Agreeing to disagree without giving up your beliefs, ideas, or ways of approaching your life takes practice and intention.

Summary

Mind is your identity and perceptions of the world. It is your concepts and how you think. Your mind is an internal, personal formation of how you make meaning of your experiences. The solar plexus reflects this energy as it engages with community and charges you to achieve goals in life. Utilizing metacognition is helpful to understand how you are thinking and perceiving. Mindfulness is a technique that can help you create space between you and your thoughts as well. The brain and central nervous system influence your mind based on neuronal patterns that fire in your brain and communicate signals to the nervous system. These patterns have been shaping you since childhood. If this is based on childhood traumas or family messages that are hurting you, employing a trauma therapist can help "rewire" these patterns.

CHAPTER 7
COMPASSION AND THE HEART CHAKRA

Loving compassion is felt strongly through the heart chakra. It is the portal to your Soul Self. When you experience a broken heart, you're feeling a disconnection from those you care for. This energy center runs deep into the ventral vagal fibers that attach to the organ of your heart. This chakra is at the "heart" of all other chakra points. When the heart chakra is clear and open, you can access the healthy forces of all other chakra points.

The color around this chakra is green, the color of growth. As green is a mixture of yellow and blue—the solar plexus below and the throat chakra above—it makes sense this chakra is a transitory energy. This chakra draws you upward and inward. The heart chakra begins your journey into the loving encounter between your human self and Soul Self. With the grounded energies of the essential chakras to act as the trunk of your human experience, the heart chakra begins your evolving spiritual one. It connects you to who you already are and to awareness beyond the earthy realms.[75]

The heart chakra has the capacity to calm. It can also heal. When clear, the heart chakra circulates Soul light through your body. Restoration ensues for the whole system with the help of

---

75. Peirce, *Frequency*, 41.

this energy. When clear, Soul light emanates outward. You then have the opportunity to spread loving connection and kindness because you are grounded in your Soul Self.

Would our world not be in a better place if we all lived more centered in our hearts?

Connection to others facilitates an understanding of what someone else is going through. This compassion, for yourself and those around you, ensures well-being.[76] This energy is always there, just waiting for you to return.

A soft alertness arises when you open to your heart chakra. You're able to settle down and be present. You can experience equanimity. This provides space for you to utilize discernment and intuition and to make honest choices. Your power lies in this deep connection to your Soul Self because this is where peace and well-being reside.

Discussing the organ that is your heart and heart chakra as it connects to our vagus nerve in this chapter will help you understand the importance of self-soothing so that you can more easily access your intuitive nature and trust your ability to determine your well-being through feeling safe on all levels.

Heart Chakra and the Vagus Nerve

Your heart is enveloped with ventral vagal nerve fibers. These fibers are faster moving, rapidly managing and sending signals throughout your system. The ventral vagal branch of the vagus nervous system manages heart rate and breathing. This nerve is linked to your cranial nerves and modulates vocal tones, speech, facial expressions, and eye movement. It helps adjust the heart's rhythm so it can

---

76. Porges, "Vagal Pathways," 189–202.

regulate, which, in turn, sends signals to your other organs that they no longer have to be on high alert.[77]

When you manage your heart rate and breath, you can calm your system. Measuring the health of the vagus nerve is done by measuring heart rate variability, or the length of time between beats. How well you can maneuver from more rapid to calmer beats is an indicator of a healthy nervous system and heart.

Determining social cues—intuiting another's state of mind—to discern whether the people are safe is imperative to your survival. As this newer part of your vagus nerve came online roughly two hundred million years ago, it helped evaluate which groups you felt safe enough to thrive in.[78] The way us mammals survive is through connection.

If the heart had its own way, it would beat rapidly all the time. To use a car metaphor, when the ventral vagus nerve gives way to the sympathetic nerve, or fight or flight responses, it's like releasing the brakes on a car when it's parked on an incline.

If you experienced complex trauma (continued trauma throughout childhood) your heart rate struggles with regulating itself. The safety messages are cross-wired because you may not be able to discern who is safe around you and who is not. According to Dr. Peter Levine, who developed a therapeutic modality called somatic experiencing ©, once trauma issues have been alleviated, the heart will return to balanced regulation.[79]

77. Porges and Dana, *Clinical Applications of the Polyvagal Theory*, 50–69.

78. Porges, *The Polyvagal Theory*, 5–6.

79. Levine, *Waking the Tiger*, 253.

EXERCISE
Be Still, My Beating Heart

This meditation derives from the polyvagal perspective mentioned above and is intended to help you notice and manage your heart rate. As always, find a safe and comfortable place to sit and alleviate distractions that are stressful.

- Notice your heart rate when you are resting. How does it feel on the in breath? On the out breath?
- Rest your palm on your heart and befriend the sensations of your heartbeats.
- Once you are feeling in sync with the beats, perform the body scan we worked through in chapter 4. Notice any tensions in your head, jaw, or neck shoulders. For each area of tension, invite the breath in to relax the tension. Continue to hold your hand to your heart and carry awareness down to your arms, back, hips, and legs. Just breathe.
- Once you are finished with the body scan, pull in a slow, regulated breath through your nose and hold it deep in your lungs for a few seconds.
- After a moment, slowly release the breath. Imagine you are blowing into a flute. Slow and deliberate.
- How do you feel? Have the beats changed?

On the exhale, your heart beats at a slower rate. When you are able to keep a measured exhale, your heart is thanking you.

Heart to Heart

Our central nervous system has a built-in need to connect with others. This is referred to as co-regulation through the polyvagal theory.[80] When we don't receive caring touch or messages of belonging growing up, we feel unprotected. The longing for connection becomes a visceral experience. Our nervous system registers a lack of security and fires off signals of danger. Minimal connection in childhood forms how we interact in relationships with intimate partners and others as adults.

Belonging is a natural instinct, and when we experience social disconnection or isolation, we develop stress symptoms. Our bodies, over time, will feel sick. Loneliness affects heart rate variability, which, in turn, affects our ability to manage a state of calm. When we feel disconnected and can't find safe people to regulate with, we reach for things outside of us to self-soothe.

Loneliness is a felt experience. So is love and belonging. Find someone you trust and connect with. Allow your nervous system to connect in laughter, safety, and friendship. Be safe and present for another and make space for the reciprocal experience of safe connection.

Chris's Story: Co-Regulation

After a decade of active military duty, Chris struggled with posttraumatic stress disorder. This had put stress on his marriage and kept him from finishing his college work, which is why he had initially called me. We had been working off and on for several years now, and when he would notice another trauma response, he would call me, and we would work through this.

---

80. Porges, *The Polyvagal Theory*, 222.

Through utilizing Eye Movement Desensitization and Reprocessing (EMDR), a good portion of his trauma responses had been alleviated or modified. Through this work, Chris had become trauma informed. He was able to recognize when his brain and central nervous system got overstimulated. He could decipher real versus perceived threats and understood what triggered them. If he had any sympathetic responses in situations that were not threatening, he could now manage them with the techniques he had learned. Chris was now working as an accountant, and he and his wife, Joanie, just bought a house.

This particular day, he came in looking tired. "Those thunderstorms killed me last night. I couldn't sleep at all." He rubbed his eyes as he sat down. "To make things worse, Joanie is out of town on a business trip this week. I paced most of the night."

"What was the worst part of the storms for you?"

"The thunder," he said. "It didn't bring on flashbacks; I just got restless. Like something was missing. I felt anxious."

We processed the response to the thunder using EMDR, then I gave him some homework.

"The weather forecast shows more storms coming tonight," I said, "so you have to snuggle with your dog."

"Huh?" he laughed.

"You know how we've talked about regulation of your vagus nervous system all these years?"

"Yeah?"

"Well, you can calm your nervous system just by being present with another's nervous system. It doesn't always have to be human, but it has to feel safe." I said. "You intuitively do this with Joanie, but she isn't in town."

"Seriously?"

"Yes," I said. "When you're tuned in and feel safe with some-one, your heart rate calms. Your dog will love the attention, and you'll be calming your sympathetic branch of your vagus nerve."

"Cool."

EXERCISE
Writing Prompt: From Five Senses to "Knowing"

Attuning to heart chakra energy is the key to feeling compas-sion for yourself and eventually others. When you do this, you are calm. When you are calm, it's a sign you're engaged in ventral vagal energy, and your body registers you are safe. You can then be safe for you and those around you. Because you're engaging in ventral vagal activity, your fight, flight, or freeze responses can take a break. Ensuring the five senses that they are safe is a good way to reach your "sixth sense" of intuitive processing.

- To begin, tune into the scents around you. Give your-self some time to notice all the layers of smell. In your journal, write down what you smell. Next to that, write down how the scents are affecting you in the moment.

- Tune into the sights around you. Notice colors, textures, the way light plays out in the space. Write down what you see. Next to that, write down how these sights are affecting you.

- Tune into your physical space. Notice how your body feels in your clothes, your chair, how the pen and journal feel. Write down the experience. Next to that, write down how these physical sensations are affect-ing you.

- Tune into the sounds around you. Be still for a while and listen carefully. Notice the sounds that are closest to you. Pay attention to sounds that may be far off in the distance. Write down what you hear. Next to that, write down how these sounds are affecting you.
- Finally, tune into the tastes you notice in your mouth. Did you just finish sipping a drink? Do you taste your last meal? Write down what you are experiencing and how you feel about it.
- Now set the journal down and tune into your heart space. Breathe deep. Let your body know it is safe. Let that sensation of safety expand through your body.

Love: The Highest Form of Compassion

The word *love* in the English language seems to send most people into various states of turmoil. *Love* is ladened with meanings of lacy hearts filled with chocolate, dopamine-induced nights, and rushing to the altar. It has also gotten entangled with highly contradictory acts, like the parent who abuses a child they are supposed to love.

Outcomes seem attached to *love* whether it's used as a noun or a verb. *Love* is the only word that connotes anything from extreme like, lust, covetousness, preferred taste in a product, fascination, overattachment to things and people, or sexually obsessed desires. *Love* gets equated with worthiness. When someone has experienced mixed messages about their lovability as a child, they grow up with complicated connections in their adult relationships. It's devastating to the psyche.

Language can be at once freeing yet limiting. What if we narrowed the definition around the word *love* to mean "value"? What comes up for you, then? Self-valuing? Valuing of others? How does that feel?

What verbs would you use in replace of *love*? *Caring*? *Honoring*? *Respecting*?

What nouns would you use in exchange of *love*? *Connection*? *Attention*?

I had a conversation once with a friend from Denmark. We were talking about the English word *love* and its overarching meanings. She shared that in Danish there are several words to describe the emotional states of love. There is a specific word that describes deep connection beyond any others. It's a word reserved only for children, spouses, or family.

Thoughtlessly, I asked her what it was.

She blushed and said, "It is a word with such intimacy, I cannot speak it in public."

Love is not simplistic, and neither is our connection to those around us. When we bond with another, the deeper aspects of us understand that we don't remain in one uncomplicated state. Love possesses degrees depending on the relationships and experiences you bring to the people you are with. Loving another has expectations, realized or not. To love is not without disappointment or frustration because peoples' realities are not always shared ones.

Loving connection with others takes an intention to hear what another's needs are and provide them, whether they are what we want or not. It takes a principled balancing act. To connect in loving ways is to hold space between two selves. It is slowing down with a need to understand yourself in the moment of connection with someone else. It's an honest assessment of self and others.

Hate: The Lowest Expression of Compassion

The word *hate* has a sophomoric quality to it. It's vicious in its simplicity. Hatred leaves no room for compassion or possibility to restore balance. Hatred takes on an either/or quality. It's a black-and-white mindset of "I am good, they are evil." It's positioning oneself as a victim in order to engage in perpetration against the person or thing being hated.

The roots of hatred are born from piety and perniciousness. Even when we have been deeply violated by another, there is an opening in our being for light and potential forgiveness. Hating keeps us from healing the harm that has been done to us.

Hatred is born of fear, and when we fear, we have lost all touch with our inner world. We are in defense mode, locked in our sympathetic nervous system. We no longer have access to our intuition and can't open to the deeper realms of our Soul. Certainly, we have cut off the opportunity of seeing another's humanness and inner light. We have shut off all possibility of grace and understanding that even the most pernicious of acts are born of someone else's fear.

When we hate, we dismiss our internal wisdom and defy awareness of the greater world. Hatred eliminates choices of healing because it is a powerless state of mind, seeking to regain itself through delivering pain to another.

People stay connected through their hatred. So do whole communities and countries. Hatred is still a bond. It's a bond we can choose or decide to break.

A Father's Compassion

One of the most powerful stories I have ever heard about the human spirit choosing healing instead of hatred is the story of Azim Khamisa. Azim could have stayed entrenched in bitterness and sought revenge for the senseless death of his son, Tariq. Instead, he heeded a richer calling within himself and discovered a level of compassion that speaks to how brilliant we can be as humans when we make the choice to forgive, which is a form of love.[81]

Azim's son, Tariq, was murdered one night in 1995. While delivering pizzas in San Diego, Tariq was shot by a fourteen-year-old boy who was part of a gang initiation. During the trial, through his shock and pain, Azim was able to see that his wasn't the only family to lose a child because of this horrific event.

He watched the fourteen-year-old boy who pulled the trigger being tried as an adult. He saw this child's family in as much pain as Azim was. Through Azim's ability to sustain the tension of grief and compassion, he reached out to the family of his son's murderer. As a result, forgiveness, compassion, and healing were able to take place. What could have been a forgotten headline from decades earlier, what could have been two families with broken hearts trapped in time, turned into a foundation that now helps prevent teen violence. In 1998, Azim founded a nonprofit organization in his son's name that mentors youth in an attempt to break the cycle of poverty and violence.[82]

What Azim did during one of the darkest times of his life was engage through compassion and the energy of his heart. Amazingly, he reached out to other human beings he could have vilified. He could have stayed in a sympathetic response that would have destroyed his health and the connection to his other loved ones for the rest of his life. Through maintaining equanimity, he reached through his pain and positively affected the outcome of people's lives forever.

---

81. Khamisa, *Azim's Bardo*.
82. "Tariq Kham-isa Foundation."

EXERCISE
Heart Chakra Connection

Perhaps the people you love are not safe, and you need to keep them at a distance. You can still wish them love and compassion. This keeps you and them in right energy by centering within yourself.

There are also times situations prevent you from joining with others you love or feel safe with. The pandemic of 2020 is an example of that. This is hard. That doesn't mean you have to feel disconnected and alone. Within you is an amazing Soul Self energy that can help you feel a deeper relationship to yourself until you can co-regulate with others again.

Try this visualization. It's intended for you to join with Soul Self energy through your heart chakra and the ventral vagus nerve.

- Breathe slowly and deeply into the heart chakra. Take as long as you need.
- Let yourself experience the expansion of energy in this area of your body.
- Feel the light inside you.
- Stay focused on the sensations in your heart. Take your time.
- Breathe into the light. This will help you feel steady and focused.
- Continue to expand that light until it's the size of your body.
- Hold the light and feel the sensation of it all around you.
- Repeat in your mind or with words, "I am enough."

Summary

Getting and receiving hugs, affirmations, being heard, and experiencing compassion is the foundation for feeling safe, hence loved. This is called co-regulating with others.

Sometimes, we can't create a safe connection with anyone, but we have the resources to help ourselves feel grounded and safe using meditation, visualization, and other exercises. This is regulation of your own system.

The heart chakra is the energy center that sends and receives love and safe connection. This area of our body unites us deeply to our own Soul Self and truth. When we can stay connected to this energy, we can emanate compassion inward to heal and outward to others. The heart chakra is the causeway to deeper, evolving aspects of who we already are as spiritual beings.

The heart is one of the organs that joins the ventral vagal nerve where we experience neurophysiological regulation. Ventral vagal engagement is the most recently developed aspect of the vagus nerve, and it assists us in knowing when we are safe with others.

CHAPTER 8
CONNECTION AND
THE THROAT CHAKRA

———•———

Only once was I blessed to physically see the color of a person's chakra. It was personally amazing. A former professor was lecturing one night. I was late for class, so I slipped into a seat on the side of the room and could only see her profile. I had just gotten back from an overseas trip that morning and was still exhilarated but also exhausted. My psychic guard was down just enough to see beyond the three-dimensional veil.

As my professor spoke, a blue mist started to emanate from her throat. I held my breath and sat forward, not daring to blink. The energy drifted up into her mouth. The more she spoke, the deeper the blue grew. After a while, her front lower jaw, up into her ears, was wrapped with a flow of indigo. Soon the whole lower section of her face and her throat were embraced in an energetic flow that, to me, showed the strength of her words in motion. What a gift I was being given.

You can probably guess from my story that indigo blue is the color surrounding the throat chakra. When you know your truth, you can speak clearly. Energy flows and you are empowered with tone and words.

Sound is fundamental for the Soul Self to express itself. The universe vibrates with sound. Our Soul Self can join with and match these frequencies.

Tone, vibration, and the words you speak affect how you co-regulate with others. Connecting through sound helps you send and receive messages of safety and caring. Your voice strengthens loving bonds and your ability to negotiate with the outside world. It soothes and heals.[83] Your voice is a herald, a call for connection. Each time you create with your voice, you allow your desires of love to manifest.[84]

Watch a child go at it with a box of crayons and paper. They are generally humming to themselves as they color. They are naturally regulating their central nervous system with their tunes, and as a result, you can feel the delight in your own system.

When you feel joy, you can express this through tone. What my professor was lecturing on that night was a healing modality she knew well and was passionate about. Her words were meant to raise our awareness so that we would one day apply this healing knowledge and spread more light into the world as therapists. Hers was a remarkable example of how this chakra has the power to reach out in a special way that none of the other chakras do.

Given its connection to the larynx and pharynx, the throat chakra sends energy outward. It calls frequencies of safe connection to those around you. It penetrates the energy of others. This energy center can be the most healing. It can also be abusive. You need to take seriously what you say as this chakra is manifesting some powerful stuff.

---

83. Goodchild, *The Naked Voice*, 53.
84. Judith and Goodman, *Creating on Purpose*, 110.

The Vagus Nerve and the Throat Chakra

We are not born with hard scales, shells, sharp teeth, or spikes on our head to keep our throat protected. Like all mammals, we rely on our group or community to keep us safe. We do this by calling out or asking for our needs to be met. It's not just what we say. It's how it is said.

The sound of someone's voice can tell us if we are welcomed long before we see the person. There is a range in our voice tone called prosody. When we are below a certain range or above it, our voice sends signals that something is wrong.[85] Low tonal ranges register signals that we might be harmed. An angry, shouting man instills fear in others. A deep thrumming registers in our nervous system that something is lurking. Doom is pending.

Think of the main theme from the 1975 movie *Jaws*, directed by Stephen Spielberg. Those first few deep notes are so familiar that anyone who hums them is jokingly telling you that danger is coming. The screeching of an ambulance's siren is not just socially conditioned to have you pay attention and move your car over to the side of the road. That high pitch plucks your sympathetic nervous system, and you look out for danger.

The one thing that confounded me when I saw my professor talking was that her throat chakra energy wasn't a perfect ball of blue circling in a clockwise or counterclockwise direction as I was taught in my yoga classes years earlier. My professor's chakric energy extended from her throat, upward into her jaw and her ears. The indigo color then ran back down into her throat the more she spoke.

---

85. Porges, *The Polyvagal Theory*, 202–214.

At the time, I didn't have a foundation in polyvagal theory as I was just a graduate student. Now, having that understanding of how we are "wired," that chakric energy flow makes sense. The network of ventral nerves fibers that connect the heart also reaches upward to the throat and into the middle ears.[86] Listening is part of speaking. Listening and speaking are part of connecting.

The energy running through the myelinated fibers of the ventral vagal branch moves fast, quickly interpreting information being sent and received. We hear meaning before it might even be spoken.

Donna Eden, in her book *Energy Medicine*, talks about the throat chakra as being the only energy center where she sees chambers on the right and left sides of the throat.[87] She says she has seen them extend upward into the brain and downward into the body and affect the body's metabolism. She writes that the right channels are anabolic and synthesize energy, while the left are catabolic and break down energy. Overlay this to the ventral vagal nerve fibers and see the correlation. The throat chakra may be the most intricate energy center in the system.

Listening is as calming to your system as speaking, and sometimes even more. When you deeply hear what someone is expressing, you are co-regulating with them. Messages of safety are sent to both central nervous systems and ventral vagal engagement begins. Your heart beats slower, and you have room in your system to connect through words and sound.

---

86. Porges, *Polyvagal Safety*, 209.
87. Eden, *Energy Medicine*, 172–73.

EXERCISE

Om Chant

Engaged ventral vagal activity in the throat and heart requires slow, deliberate release on an exhale. The "Om" chant, the chant you hear Buddhist monks repeating, is a sound that comes from deep within your diaphragm and is guided up through your lungs and out your throat.

By utilizing the diaphragmatic muscles, then the vagal nerve fibers in your mouth, jaw, and throat, you are centering your body. You also clear your root, sacral, solar plexus, heart, and throat chakras for a more compassionate connection. Think: upward, then outwards.

The chant is also a calming resonance for others to hear. The sound naturally falls into a midrange tonally. It is said "Om" is the sound of the universe.

The "Om" chant has four separate parts, or measures, to the chant. The first is the "A" (ah) sound. The second is the "U" (ooh) sound. The first two sounds of "A" and "U" meld into a long "O" sound that creates a humming effect with your mouth open.

Go ahead and try this.

The third measure is the "M." It is not a clipped consonant at the end. The "M" leads to a long, soft drop-off. Think of this as a soft hum with the mouth closed. Let this whole sound release until your lungs have been emptied of air. Then breathe deeply and express this sound again.

Compassionate Connection: That Two-Way Street We're On

Listening deeply is truly one of the greatest gifts you can give another person. You must want to connect to hear, which is a loving gesture in itself. Even more than speaking, listening takes intention to slow down and be present. This shows the other person that you care enough to honor their perspective.

Compassionate, loving energy fills a room when you are together in honorable, forthright ways. When you listen, you are saying through body language that you respect, honor, value, and perhaps love this person enough to be available to them. If a person is not perceived as safe, you would neither face them nor meet their gaze. Your body would be on guard. There is a natural measure of security in the connection when you can face them.

Even in a work environment—where personal vulnerability isn't the objective—there needs to be intention to listen. You are sharing ideas and constructs with each other. There is a shared outcome with coworkers, and for that to be obtained, a healthy connection needs to be in place. Coworkers who are not feeling safe within themselves enough to be present to another can really wreak havoc in a meeting. Sound familiar?

When you enter into any dialogue, you show that you are willing to connect. Having good ventral vagal tone during these times opens the heart and throat chakras. Even in business negotiations, this is your power source. With this energy comes clarity, and you can extend yourself without (or with less) anxiety or fear. For your words to have any value, you need to be clear and true about what you say. This creates honest and open dialogue, whether in a personal or impersonal setting. True dialogue requires honesty. A lack of truth in the words you speak creates a contaminated experience.

In his best-selling book *The Four Agreements*, Don Miguel Ruiz discusses the first of these four agreements you choose to live by as being impeccable with your word.[88] What does that mean to you? How can you speak from clarity, kindness, and truth? This takes intention and consistency to apply such a principle. It may take time for you to believe you can be impeccable with your word. What would it feel like to have others see you as someone who was always honest with what you say?

No matter the type of relationship, how you use your words—what you say to another—matters.

Responding: Highest Expression of Connection

There was a picture of Bishop Desmond Tutu and the Dalai Lama circulating the internet shortly after Bishop Tutu died in 2021. The bishop is reaching out to affectionately squeeze the Dalai Lama's lips and jaw as the Dali Lama is about to kiss the bishop. This image of two of the most famous spiritual leaders of our time feeling intimate enough to joke around each other's face and mouths struck me. This is compassionate connection at its highest intention. To allow someone close to your mouth and throat takes deep-rooted trust. The throat and mouth are the most vulnerable yet expressive parts of your body.

Reliability and the intention to be accountable to the other person for how you say or do something is at the heart of responding. A response needs to be thought through with the understanding that your words and gestures affect the people you're in communication with. Response is an intention to communicate toward a compassionate outcome. It's about creating resolution, not conflict.

---

88. Ruiz, *Four Agreements*, 25.

Dialogue at its finest.

Compassionate responses require you to take that moment between what is said and done by another and what you say or do. When you can do this, you are in your authentic Self and utilizing ventral vagal activation like a finely tuned instrument.

Responding also has at its core healthy boundaries. Effective boundary setting honors another person's perspective—even if you don't agree—without losing a handle on yours. In chapter 5, "Emotions and the Sacral Chakra," I gave two examples of how to communicate in ways that honor both you and another. Those examples are always great to revisit.

Boundary setting begins with a pause. A breath. An intention.

Reacting: Lowest Expression of Compassion

Reaction comes from a defensive place. It isn't thought through, and its aim is to dominate and defend. Examples of reacting would be yelling or screaming, using hurtful names or language, mocking, gossiping, or ignoring the individual. All these gestures are done from a position of perceived powerlessness.

Words mean very little if they are not spoken or heard with the intention of honest connection. Being talked at or "verbal diarrhea" are attempts to control or manage anxiety. This is just an overreactive engagement with your sympathetic nervous system. It's an exercise in tension release at someone else's expense. Monologue is not dialogue.

The energy from the throat chakra can be abused with the objective to steal another's power. When words are used in this way, you twist yours and others' energy centers. You absorb the karma of the ones you are attempting to hurt since, through words, you are trying to add to their pain.

Another example of a reaction is being belligerent to a boss, colleague, or person in a position of authority. It also works the other way by attempting to abuse someone with less authority than you. This is aggression. It's not thought out. It's an immature, pugnacious retort that induces a shot of cortisol into the system. For a moment, you feel superior to someone, but in the long run, you have given your power away. Reason comes from the higher levels of your brain. Reactivity comes from the middle emotional brain that activates the fight or flight response.

How often have you been able to remain calm and present to someone shouting at you? The answer is probably never since it's nearly impossible to do so. Your central nervous system registers the loud high frequencies of someone's voice as dangerous. Someone yelling is also activating frequencies of domination in your chakras and auras that are going to affect you energetically.

This is common ground that gets covered in family or couple's sessions I have with clients. Someone is mad when the other person walks away from a raised voice. The person raising their voice is not feeling heard and falls into a domination pattern with their voice. The other person has a fired up nervous system that can only be managed by leaving the situation.

Both people are fearfully activated, whether they know it or not. One feels rejected, the other feels attacked. Sound familiar?

Another form of reaction is more pernicious and calculated. It's countering your own disowned feelings by gossiping or character assassinating other people. It manipulates the chakras and central nervous system of the person you are gossiping with too. It's a power-over attempt not just to hurt the person being talked about but to manipulate the person's energy you are gossiping with. Anything that creates a subversive negative effect is a reactive response.

EXERCISE
Tapping the Energy Through

The exercise of tapping is known to some as emotional focus technique (EFT) and to others as energy psychology (EP). It is also called acupoint tapping. There are some minor differences between the three, but they are essentially all the same.

This modality has been studied extensively for its efficacy in alleviating stress in a person's system.[89] I use the technique in my own practice to show clients how to self-soothe when they are home. Tapping can be done inside or outside a clinician's office, but I would always caution not to process your own traumatic memories alone.

Tapping is based on the ancient Chinese practice of acupuncture but would be considered acupressure. Acupuncture applies needles to the meridians and other energy centers in the body, while acupressure applies pressure to these areas. Meridians are different from the chakras. Using our car analogy, chakras are the lights that beam outward, while meridians are the "wiring" that carry the energy throughout the vehicle. Utilizing tapping techniques employs the energy in the meridians.

I have found tapping to be a fabulous resource for helping people self-soothe. One of the reasons I put this exercise in this chapter is because the nerve fibers along the throat and face are near these pressure points. Tapping can be easily learned. How you use tapping here is to help engage the ventral vagus nerve and balance the chakras and etheric energies.

Examine figure 4 and notice where the dots are. They are placed at the crown chakra, the third eye chakra, at the edges

---

89. Feinstein, Eden, and Craig, *The Promise of Energy Psychology*, 78.

of the eyes, below the eyes, under the nose, and under the lower lip. There are two more at the area of the chest below the breastbone (next to the heart chakra) and two on the sides of the ribs. This is the order you will tap in, starting with the crown chakra.

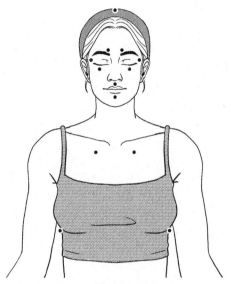

Figure 4: Tapping Exercise

Take a moment and tap on each of these acupoints for practice. Now we want to combine this tapping with a belief system or state of mind that is not serving you. Follow these steps:

1. What is a state of being that troubles you right now? Are you tired, scared, anxious, overwhelmed, depressed, angry, or sad? Any state of mind you're struggling with will do.
2. Rate the intensity of this experience on a scale from 0 to 10.

3. Fill in the blank in this statement:
   "Even though I am _____, I deeply and completely accept myself." You don't have to agree with
   self-acceptance. Just trust in this process.

4. Start tapping from the crown chakra and repeat the
   statement. When you have finished the statement,
   move on to the next pressure points, tapping and
   repeating the statement until you have gone through
   each pressure point.

5. Repeat step 4 three times.

6. Now check in with your body. Is your intensity scale
   above zero? If so, continue tapping until you have no
   more charge in your body.

Overactive Throat Chakra

Like any chakra, the throat chakras can be too open. Signs that your
throat chakra lacks boundaries are:

- Monologuing
- Shouting or talking over others
- Inability to stop talking around people
- Sharing inappropriate information about yourself or
  others
- Inappropriate or mean comments to others
- Gossiping about others
- Verbal abuse
- Judging
- Mocking or making sounds meant to humiliate

These are also issues related to emotional boundaries since
expressing emotions is primarily a verbal process. Anxiety and

overactivity with the sympathetic nervous system can create an imbalance in ventral vagal activity. Working through anxiety, calming the body, and putting focus on ventral vagal safety in the body can help.

True reflection on how you are thinking and psychological insight is another way to find balance with this energy center. This chakra is not a separate entity to be soothed. It is a result of many other factors of how people engage in their lives.

Underactive Throat Chakra

Do you remember a time you were upset and wanted to speak but the constriction in your throat made it difficult? Is this a regular pattern for you? When you have been told that your opinion doesn't matter, you struggle with asking for what you need. Some signs of an underactive throat chakra are:

- Pain or constriction in throat, chest, jaw, and even neck
- "I don't know" statements
- Passive-aggressive statements
- Not owning up to things you have said
- Problems with swallowing
- Issues with nasal passages
- Inability to speak up for yourself or others
- Flat prosody and weak-sounding voice
- Not being honest with self or others
- Fear statements

The struggle to use words can be deeply ingrained in your nervous system because of a lack of safety from childhood. If you dissociated to get through chaos or abuse, these neuronal patterns are ingrained, and it will be difficult to speak up during stressful situations as an adult. Surrounding yourself with safe people who will listen, defining how you are feeling and thinking and what you want to say can help. Engaging in ventral vagal safety is key as this will begin to repattern the messages in your system.

EXERCISE
Writing Prompt: Forgiveness Prayer

Have you heard of the Ho'oponopono chant? It is an ancient Hawaiian practice of healing by taking full responsibility for your actions or words.

In your journal, write the names of anyone you believe you have hurt in the past because of your words. Speak their name before you recite the following chant:

I'm sorry,
please forgive me,
thank you,
I love you.

Summary

Listening is part of speaking and connection through a polyvagal perspective. The network of vagal nerve fibers that connects the heart and lungs reach upward to the throat, larynx, and into the middle ears, making the energy around the throat chakra a powerful source of soothing and connection. The energy running through these myelinated fibers moves quickly, interpreting information being sent and received.

Throat chakra energy is powerful. It is the only energy that is generated outward in a deliberate attempt to connect with or hurt others. Our throat resonates sounds. It is through the sound of language that you can ask for your needs to be met.

CHAPTER 9
SPIRITUALITY AND THE THIRD EYE CHAKRA

———————•———————

The third eye chakra is located just above the bridge of your nose between the brows. It's associated with purple—the royal color. Utilizing the energy of the "mind's eye" brings you deeper into your internal uniqueness. It connects you to the symbolic, energetic, and nonphysical aspects of who you already are.[90]

In human form, you have a natural inclination to define, categorize, and classify. Your left brain helps you create with others and be part of a common language. Cultures and security are established with linear and measurable concepts. Where you get into trouble is when you neglect your immeasurable internal experiences that are seen through the third eye chakra. Denying these encounters because they don't match up with the outer world doesn't mean the information and messages aren't of value or real. Accepting that your experiences will not fit neatly into the messages of the outside world is part of embracing your spirituality.

The third eye chakra is where your human form symbolically meets your Soul Self. Classifying a Soulful experience is impossible since words are limited in this inner realm. You cannot measure these experiences; you can only be present to them. Your Soul is

———————————————

90. Peirce, *Frequency*, 40.

an energy that's in constant transformation. It knows no limits because it has no limits. Utilizing the energy of your third eye puts you into an encounter with acceptance. Being present to information not readily available to your logical mind is its own form of spiritual maturity.

Utilizing the third eye chakra plays a role in what the prefrontal cortex of your brain is already doing: calming, managing, and looking for a bigger picture. The perceptions you receive from this chakra can play a reassuring role throughout your whole body as you heal a lifetime of harsh experiences and the effects they had on you.

Third Eye Chakra and the Vagus Nerve

Third eye chakra energy runs through your prefrontal cortex. This part of the brain conceptualizes, theorizes, and comprehends a richer meaning to situations. The ventromedial portion of the prefrontal cortex is what creates your capacities to understand the abstract, feel connection to other humans, and even intuit future outcomes.[91] This higher reasoning section of your brain links with the survival segments of your body, such as the amygdala and brain stem. With these multimodal sensory connections in place, your more rational prefrontal cortex can modulate impulsive behaviors coming from the "survival portions" of your nervous system.

The pituitary gland, the thalamus, and the hypothalamus are part of the axis that regulates hormone "messaging" in your body. These glands rest between the left and right portions of your prefrontal cortex behind the bridge of the nose. They are the pinnacle of the hypothalamic-pituitary-adrenal (HPA) and

91. Kawasaki and Reddy, "Investigation of Human Cognition in Epilepsy Surgery Patients."

hypothalamic-pituitary-gonadal (HPG) axes that connect and send signals to and from your vagus nervous system. Hormonal output sends signals through your nervous system.

Remember that the right and left vagus nerves have different regulatory functions, just as the brain does.[92] In overly simplified terms, one works more intuitively, while one works more linearly. Nerve fibers intricately connect your eyes to your brain and vagus nerve. Eye movements, which you do naturally in your sleep with rapid eye movement (REM) while dreaming, stimulate blood flow to the vagus nerve and send information throughout your system.

The Eyes Are the Window to Your Soul—and Your Vagus Nerve

Your eye movement is a lot less random than you think. Your eyes naturally process information based on where they are looking. Noticing where your eyes move to and what they sometimes lock onto helps increase awareness of what is occurring emotionally for you. This can also help you understand how to move your eyes so you can work through life matters as they arise.

Have you ever watched someone else's eyes while they were talking? Did their eyes glance up or search the room while they were trying to find an answer to a question? Did they look back and forth as they explored an emotion or an impactful memory? Your whole system is receiving and processing the information it needs on a regular basis, and your eyes are an integral part in this.

Over the last several decades, research has shown the movement of your eyes plays an important role in emotional processing. This is how therapeutic modalities such as Eye Movement

---

92. Porges, *The Polyvagal Theory*, 135.

Desensitization and Reprocessing (EMDR) and expansions of this modality, such as brainspotting, developed.[93] Eye movement techniques are well-researched ways for therapists to help their clients work traumatic responses out of their system. As more research shows that trauma can't just be talked through, more body/mind modalities are developed and employed in therapy.[94] Therapeutic approaches have become far more intrinsic to all the dimensions of self, which leads to more rapid, long-term healing.

EXERCISE
Soft Gazing

Here's a technique I learned that engages both the physical sight and third eye vision. The exercise was shown to me years ago by an intuitive energy reader, and it employs some of the relaxing ways we utilize our eyes to alleviate stressors.

This exercise will help you read the energy of living things. It's also a very calming process for the central nervous system and a great example of how calming the central nervous system helps us employ access to our more intuitive nature. These are skills we can all develop. Let's see how you experience this exercise.

- As always, get comfortable in your sacred space and take in a few deep breaths.
- Find a plant near you. This could be a tree outside your window, flowers in your garden, or a house plant. If you

---

93. Shapiro, *Eye Movement Desensitization and Reprocessing (EMDR)*. Grand, *Brainspotting*.
94. Ogden, Minton, and Pain, *Trauma and the Body*, 4.

don't have plants in your house, consider this the next time you are at a store with plants.

- Look at the center of the plant. Just gaze.
- As you stare at the center of the plant, utilize your peripheral vision. Keep your eyes on the center of the plant.
- Notice if you see any color, movement, or shapes on the outer rim of the plant.
- Don't try to figure anything out. Just gaze.
- You can do this for as long as you like. You can repeat the exercise as many times as you would like as well.

Eyes on the Prize

Employing the eyes in any self-soothing strategies is powerful since this will initiate both exteroceptive and interceptive awareness.[95] If you relax or close your eyes, you're regulating a natural reflex called the oculocardiac reflex. This engages arterial baroceptors that send a calming response to your central nervous system and manage blood pressure.

When you're tired, do you find yourself gazing out the window or just staring at a spot in the room? Staring is a common physiological stress reliever.

While staring and softening your gaze are calming, activating your eyes can also bring tremendous relief to your body. Your intuitive third eye will engage in the process as images, information, or a knowing about things arise. This is a powerful method. I call it "stretching the eyes." Didn't know you could do that, did you?

95. Marshall et al., "Exteroceptive Expectations Modulate Interoceptive Processing."

Just like a muscle stretch, this process may at first bring discomfort since it's releasing congested energy. If you stay with it, though, then just like a muscle stretch, you'll get that relaxing sensation. When stretching is associated with the eyes and the brain, you may be releasing stored emotions, so it's important to know when you are asking too much of yourself or if you need professional help doing this.

While most of us can't imagine rolling our eyeballs around until we find relief, it actually helps. The eyes are attached to your vagus nerve, so when you do this, you may also feel a "stretch" in the form of stimulation or activation in your body that doesn't make sense. Sometimes, the activation occurs on the opposite side of your body from where you are looking. This is a good thing. Know that you are listening to what your body tells you despite how weird or self-conscious you may initially feel.

I have done this in my own personal therapy sessions, and it has alleviated some very interesting physiological and emotional responses. I will also do this at home—no matter how silly I might look to my family—if I'm feeling the need for it. The following section is an eye stretching exercise.

EXERCISE
Stretching the Eyes

Before you perform this exercise, know that you should listen to your body. If you have any medical ailments that make this exercise uncomfortable, do not do this. Track the physiological and emotional messages this process brings out. Trust your own intuition. See how this exercise works for you.

You will definitely need to sit down. Get comfortable for this exercise. Choose a safe place where you can sit securely. As always, center yourself with your breaths for a moment. I would recommend closing your eyes, as this will activate third eye intuition. There is no time frame for this; just gauge when you've had enough. The information you get may be richer as a result. However, if you feel safer keeping your eyes open, you will still receive the benefits from this exercise.

1. Roll your eyes around.
2. As you roll your eyes, find a point where your eyes seem to want to stay.
3. Let them stay there for a while. Breathe.
4. Notice, as your eyes stay put, what is changing in your central nervous system?
5. Hold this "stretch" until you feel relief or a shift in your body.

Reception: Highest Expression of Spirituality

Receiving and accepting the energy that presents to you is the most spiritual thing you can do. Trusting the symbolic, etheric information that flows as you open to your inner world is hard. It takes restraint not to push away impressions or go look something up that you have no reference for. It's our nature to want to categorize a metaphysical experience. Messages from deep within are beyond the third dimension. If you were raised in a religious environment, the symbols and religious direction came from outside of you. It takes time to trust what's coming from within.

Embrace your light. This is where your Soul resides. The deeper you can listen to what your intuitive essence is telling you, the deeper you can understand your Soul. With spirituality, there's no duality. There is no theology. There is no either/or comparison and no absolutes. Spirituality is fluid because it's a connection to who you already are.

Awareness of your internal experience takes holding space for yourself and trusting. Accepting that your reality will vary from another's inner truths leaves room within you to go deeper and stay open. Just like we've been talking about boundaries around your body, emotions, thoughts, and words, there are boundaries around your own internal experience. This is your private, inner world. It doesn't have to match up with what others believe you should feel and believe. At times, the connection to your inner world can be so unique you might feel alone. This is not necessarily a collective experience. Give your inner work time to grow. Your journey back to Soul Self requires alone time to reconnect. This is where your sacred space comes in handy.

Bypassing: Lowest Expression of Spirituality

Spiritual bypassing is an attempt to connect to the higher realms without being willing to heal past wounds that stemmed from childhood.[96] Exclusively focusing on spiritual transformation, elevation, or developing certain psychic abilities without healing your painful childhood is a distortion of self. When you don't reflect and heal old patterns, you work from blind spots that repeat. It's like a top-heavy tree with a narrow, soft trunk that will eventually tip over.

Continual pursuit of the energy "high" in spiritual practice can lead to trouble when it's an attempt to avoid those rocky areas we must all circle back around to for healing. A quest for an exclusive inner world with no connection to others is avoidance.

---

96. Fossella, "Human Nature, Buddha Nature."

The self-identification from the solar plexus chakra—those strongholds of mind and personality that we cling to in this world—can override and distort the spiritual messages we get in our third eye chakra if we're not aware of this. Third eye energy can drive your ego.

If you deny family patterns that were hurtful and continue to repeat unhealthy relationships, you're just retraumatizing yourself. The third eye chakra can get abused when people don't want to do the healing work because it might require physical discomfort. Spiritual bypassing does nothing to help ensure growth and healing. It's a parlor trick.

Susan's Story: When Spiritual Bypassing No Longer Works

Susan canceled two appointments with me before she finally came in. She had been working with energy healers, hypnotherapists, and bodyworkers and made it clear—therapy wasn't her thing. Her constant relapsing with her addiction to pain pills and acting out sexually with men she was meeting online had put her in the hospital. She had been physically assaulted by a strange man she met to have sex with.

Even then, she made it clear she felt she could handle her addiction through meditation and bodywork. Of course, I didn't disagree with this. Meditation was not enough to "fix" the reason she wanted to escape with pills and high-risk sex in the first place. Her only reason for coming to see me was because she had been put on probation for possession of illegal drugs. Losing family support and her third Narcotics Anonymous sponsor, experiencing an assault, and being told by her doctor she had to get serious or her addiction would kill her had not been the final straws to help herself. She just didn't want to go to jail. She stated that coming to a therapist was her last option.

"How long do you think therapy will take?" she asked.

"Honestly? As long as it takes," I said. "It truly depends since addiction covers a lot of deeper issues that have to be worked through slowly."

"I was hoping this would take about three or four visits."

"Months, maybe years," I said. "If you truly want to stabilize your life. Therapy is just one of the ways you need to do that."

It took several months for Susan to trust me enough to share she had been repeatedly molested by the next-door neighbor as a child. We worked through helping her identify her trauma responses and discovered what triggered them. Susan dissociated to the point that she lost time in her body. This was happening more frequently now since she was having to regularly face her perpetrator.

Susan's mother, who still lived in the house Susan grew up in, had suffered a stroke during my work with Susan. Susan had to go back to the house regularly because she was her mother's only care-taker. This meant Susan was continually being retraumatized. In the early part of our work, that also meant Susan was struggling with staying clean despite her regular drug testing under court supervision.

Susan went back into Narcotics Anonymous and attended daily meetings. She struggled enough that she stated she wanted to attend residential treatment so she could help stabilize her cravings. In the meantime, Susan found in-home healthcare support for her mother, so she wasn't regularly going to the old house.

After she left residential treatment, she said she felt stable enough to process her trauma. We utilized EMDR and other somatic processing modalities. We worked in ways that spoke to

Susan's natural curiosity for the metaphysical. I helped her understand the emotional signals in her chakras so she could make meaning from her current experiences of what was happening in her body. She could soon ground enough in her body to be present during difficult conversations with people. This brought her more seriously into her yoga practice as she wanted to explore the sensations of being grounded.

Because Susan had done so much previous work with yoga, meditation, and the chakras, she wasn't intimidated to reattend her old groups. Now that Susan was sober and clearheaded, she said she was surprised by just how much information and insight she hadn't pulled in during those years of attending classes while high.

"I can really feel a stretch in my body during an asana now," she said, "and meditation is so real. Before I was just dissociated and thinking I had it going on because I wasn't there."

"You're learning your body is safe now, aren't you?"

For Susan, her struggle was complex enough that it took three years to feel fully grounded and be in solid recovery. She has been clean for years now, working a strong program, and has completed her yoga teaching certification. She understands now that while everything she was seeking to do on a spiritual level was good, she was doing it only to stay feeling good.

Ways We Bypass

It is my personal belief that if we didn't spend so much time and energy running from what we perceive as emotional pain, we would be a more loving, present world in general. Spiritual practices are not the only ways to build fortresses around our "soft spots." Here are just a few more ways we employ coping strategies that push back emotion:

- Drugs, alcohol, and addictive processes
- Denial (This could be about your family history of abuse, insisting it hasn't affected you, not wanting to notice patterns of bad relationships, etc.)
- Avoiding anger, sadness, or any emotions perceived as difficult
- Blocking childhood memories (This may be a form of survival and disconnection that started early in life.)
- Avoiding therapy
- Blaming others
- Refusing to examine and take responsibility for your own aggressive or passive-aggressive behaviors
- Isolating to the point of depression
- Rescuing others
- Controlling outcomes, especially with other people
- Spending most of your free time meditating and not relating to others
- Being the healer without doing the healing for yourself
- Stopping therapy when you're on the cusp of working through emotional issues because it makes you uncomfortable
- Fear of intimacy and vulnerability by avoiding connection with others

Reflect a moment on how you push back against more complicated emotions or if what appear to be emotions are physiological responses from old hurts. I would also suggest that you use your journal as a place to write down what you're feeling and where you're feeling it. If you see the more painful emotions as your Soul simply asking to be heard, does this make it easier for you to be present to yourself?

The Psychological Is the Spiritual

Please don't misinterpret my meaning in the previous sections. I wouldn't be writing a book like this if I believed that spiritual practices of meditation, yoga, energy work, mediumship, or past-life or life-between-life regression work aren't amazing healing components. These explorations into our psyche lead to a lifetime commitment of healthy balance and understanding of a deeper way of being. However, when you use these methods to dissociate from emotional pain and psychological wounding from early childhood, you're using the spiritual work as an addiction—a way to numb.

This is why counseling to help with trauma and how you learned to attach to loved ones early on is vital. When you work through the denser issues and old memories that recirculate through your nervous system and brain, you clear up those energetic strongholds that keep you from feeling safe and loved. When you can do this, spirituality is naturally integrated into your life.

Spirituality should have no narrative beyond the experience of connecting to your internal world. The Tibetans call the concept *nangba*. The Christian mystics called it Gnostic. The Jewish faith refers to it as Kabbalah. These are all words that denote a mystical, spiritual knowing or turning inward for connection. Regardless of which journey and which interpretation you accept, connecting inward is connecting higher. Let's do some work, utilizing your eye movement to connect to your third eye chakra.

EXERCISE
Third Eye Connection

You utilize the third eye every day. Each time you imagine or see something that "doesn't make sense," you're engaging this intuitive, sensing aspect. Third eye seeing isn't something in addition to your physical sight; it is intertwined with all your other senses. If trusted, third eye chakra energy allows you the experience of individuation. Practice connecting to what you already know.

- Sit with spine straight but not tense.
- Close your eyes for a while and connect with your breath.
- Gaze up to the point between your eyes where your third eye chakra is.
- Breathe through your nostrils and feel the sensation of the air as it fills the upper chamber of your sinuses.
- Continue to focus on this area of your body.
- Allow yourself several minutes to sit.
- Notice how your energy shifts. Do any symbols, shapes, colors, or information come to you?

Spirit Guides and Ancestors: They Are There For You

We do not walk this world alone. Even in your most lonely of times, you have the loving support of community from realms you cannot see with the physical eye.[97] Those who stand by you and support your time on this earth plane are loved ones who have passed, those from soul groups you don't remember in this life, or angelic beings. Even if you have had poor attachment to loved ones on this earth plane, you can take comfort in knowing those who watch over you are doing so in love and support.[98] What behaviors they might have possessed during their time on earth have

---

97. Cannon, *Between Death and Life*, 50.
98. Newton, *Destiny of Souls*, 16.

transformed in their crossing. Their intentions evolve into love and empathy because that's what the spirit realm is. The love and support from them is vast and beyond understanding in human form.

The most generous thing you can do for yourself is accept that you're cared for and watched over, even when you can't fully comprehend this. Once you allow this connection of love, you will never feel alone or unsupported again.

Through the use of your third eye chakra, you can connect to the unseen realms of spirit and your guides. Have confidence in the information the energy sources give to you. Since the realm of spirit is of a higher frequency, the information the third eye provides is refined.[99] Regular meditation can be a powerful process to access this world.

EXERCISE
Grounding and Shielding

Anytime we reach into the spirit realm, we need to take time to ground and protect our energy. This exercise will help do that before we establish connection. Your intention is not to draw to you just any energies, but the ones that guide you. Consider this like looking for your best friends in a public place. There is usually more than one person who will notice you, or maybe even want to say something to you. You want to be with the ones who watch over you and help you feel safe.

Connection beyond the veil takes practice. Some are more comfortable with this. Some have a natural inclination to it; however, everyone can do this. This is not a parlor trick; this is reaching out for guidance, love, protection, and direction in life.

---

99. Cannon, *Between Death and Life*, 50.

We all have this "wiring" to connect. It just gets dismissed so frequently that we become skeptical.

Nature is a fantastic place for grounding and peace if you have access. The energies around trees and natural areas will embrace you and filter out distractions. If you can't be outside, your sacred space is fantastic. When I'm in mine, I like to pull the four elements of this world into my meditations. I use a candle (fire), diffuser (water), and plants and rocks (earth). These clear the fourth element, air, for me.

Utilizing your five bodily senses of sight, smell, sound, touch, and taste is important for grounding. This helps you stay connected to your own energy before you engage the sixth sense accessed by your third eye. I believe as we connect to spirit, we need to stay established in our physical realm. This is a step many people dismiss, and as a result, they can get dissociated and unknowingly reach for things like excessive amounts of food to ground.

One more note: put your journal and writing implements to the side of you; you may want to reach for them after this experience.

- As you settle in, apply your sight. Notice the colors, textures, patterns, and shapes of your environment. If these are familiar to you, see them differently. One way to do this is to observe how the light is casting patterns.
- Take in a deep breath. First for grounding, then for connection to your space. Notice the scents in the air. Have you used any essential oils? As you attune to smells, how do you experience your space differently?

- Now just listen. Take some time to truly hear. What are the more obvious daily sounds around you that you might normally filter out? Are there sounds way off in the distance? Are you in a familiar place but hearing things you didn't notice before?
- Gently move your fingers, then rest them on your lap. What do you feel? These movements are familiar, but make an attempt to experience them differently.
- Shift the attention to your mouth. Notice what you are tasting. Is it this afternoon's lunch? Gum? Let yourself be aware without judgment. We carry taste in our mouth but generally don't pay much attention to it. How does this help to ground you?
- Through the experience of your third eye, imagine a soft, iridescent, shimmering rain encircling you or filling the room. This is an energy of protection and clearing. Let yourself adjust to its softness and the feelings of calm it brings. You are safe.
- Recite a soft invocation to state intention. Here is one: "The guides and information that come to me are for the highest and wisest purpose."
- Continue connection with third eye energy. Notice what images, shapes, colors, or messages you receive internally. Just observe. The information may not make sense to your brain because it is being expressed in figurative ways. Symbolism and what we consider our imagination are the language of spirit and your Soul Self.
- Ask for one of your guides to step forward. Hold the space for the experience. Ask questions and see what the responses are.

- When you are done, thank your guides and reconnect to your five senses and the elements in your physical space.

EXERCISE
Writing Prompt: Intuitive Writing

This prompt has no firm rules because it is exclusive to your inner experience and awareness. After the above meditation, break out your journal and colored pencils, crayons, or markers.

Close your eyes and connect with the energy of your third eye. Draw your experience.

Another way to approach this is to keep your journal on hand as you connect with your guides. As you see images and color more clearly, with eyes closed, draw them. Ask your guides questions. Write the responses on paper. The more you do this, the easier the flow will become for you.

Summary

Our journey inward with the third eye chakra places us directly into ventral vagal activity. These nerve fibers connect with the eyes, and your eyes play an important role in emotional processing. Therapeutic modalities such as EMDR developed with this understanding. Eye movement techniques are well-researched ways for therapists to help their clients work traumatic responses out of their system.

Trust that we also have an intuitive third eye, which leads us to deeper Soul Self truths. With that understanding, be open to what this third eye reveals to you. It is true—your eyes are a window to your Soul.

CHAPTER 10
EMPATHY AND THE CROWN CHAKRA

The crown chakra rests at the very top of your head. It is the link upward into the universal realms and flows downward into your body. This chakra is a reminder that we are all divinely linked to a universal web of compassion. This is where empathy lies, with the understanding we are all working through this experience of being human.

Consider the crown chakra energy like a spiritual outlet. You can plug in and refuel divine light into your system. Through this chakra you transform. When you're open to it, the crown chakra offers your system brilliant messages.[100] The downloads you get are exclusive to your needs and carry light and love. This energy center is a sort of heavenly co-regulation experience, if you will.

This is also an energetic center that can be easily overlooked, especially as you go about the stressors in your daily life. I will notice that as I begin to think, read, or utilize my left-brain intellectual activities, my crown chakra closes up and I have to make an effort to reconnect to it.

Those who don't utilize their crown chakra tend to pull vitality from others in an unconscious attempt to get their emotional

---

100. Judith, *Eastern Body, Western Mind*, 392–97.

needs met. The crown chakra is like the lodestone in a compass. A lodestone is drawn to the magnetic forces in the earth's pole. The crown chakra affects and can improve your health because it links to a source of divine energy. It can be accessed through simple meditation and focus to improve spiritual well-being.[101]

Universal Source, that web of light that unites all Souls, is where empathy lies. The relationship to something greater helps us to understand we are all connected.

Violet is the color of the crown chakra. Saint Germain's healing illumination is violet. There can be no mistaking the overlay here. For centuries, mystics have opened to Saint Germain's violet light for balancing, restoring, and eliminating energies that no longer serve them. So can you. When you're depleted, the crown chakra is your generator.

Crown Chakra and the Vagus Nerve

The crown chakra sits at the center of your skull and resides between the prefrontal lobe and the parietal lobe. The energy aligns with the circle of Willis, where the major arteries at the base of the brain run.[102] The left and right branches of the vagus nerve start here, in cranial nerve X.

This area of the brain is also where the afferent fibers of the ophthalmic nerve, trigeminal nerve, and maxillary nerve and the mandibular nerve begin.[103] All these nerve fibers are what send sensations back and forth from your face to your brain and provide the abilities for smell, sight, eye movement, taste, hearing, and balance. The nerve activity at the top of the brain, which is also

---

101. Weiss, *Directing Our Inner Light*, 16.
102. Carter et al., *The Human Brain Book*, 43.
103. Porges, *The Polyvagal Theory*, 288.

where the crown chakra is, embarks you on your human encounter with the world by helping you engage with the five senses.

As we mentioned in chapter 9, the upper portion of the brain generates higher reasoning and imaginal, symbolic, and intuitive functioning. Both the crown chakra and the third eye chakra are also connected to the dorsal medial nucleus in the thalamus, which acts like a filter from the brain stem.[104] This area of the thalamus relays emotional and sensory messages and messages of sleep and consciousness to the prefrontal cortex. As we have been discussing with the evolving chakras, the afferent nerves along the throat, third eye, and crown chakra are where we listen, gather, and communicate emotional connection and higher awareness. This is the need to be understood and to understand others—the root of empathy.

EXERCISE
Ventral Vagal and Crown Chakra Connection

You can never underestimate the healing power of your own touch when you need to regulate yourself. The energy centers in the palms of your hands carry loving heart chakra energy down your arms and outward.[105] Your head is a delicate feature of your body despite the heavy lifting it does for you. Soothing by using your hands to cradle the energy centers on your head and face can give you a sense of loving connection to yourself.

104. Carter et al., *The Human Brain Book*, 180.
105. Kunz and Krieger, *The Spiritual Dimensions of Therapeutic Touch*, 133.

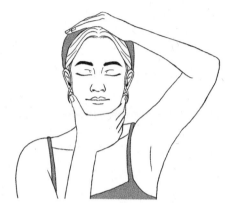

Figure 5: Soothing the Crown and Vagus

- Place your choice of hand on the lower portion of your jaw. Your chin should rest nicely in the crux of your thumb and index finger with your palm facing toward your throat chakra.
- Rest your other hand, palm down, on the top of your skull at the crown chakra.
- Once you settle into this position, draw in a breath.
- Now slowly and fully exhale, engaging that ventral vagal activity and lowering your heart rate on the out breath.
- Breathe like this for a long as you need to settle.

In this exercise, the fingers on the lower portion of your jaw rest nicely on the myelinated nerves that line your face, neck, and middle ear. The palms of your hands have their own chakric energy, and all of these energy centers, from your head and hands, are connected in a nice circulating flow that sends safety cues through your vagus nerve and chakras.

With the hand on your chin, you're gently stimulating the ventral vagal nerve fibers around your face and neck. See this hand as cradling your face. How does that feel? Stay in this position for as long as you want. After using your hands in one way, switch hands. See how this new positioning feels. Does the energy change as you change your hands? Do this anytime you need to feel safe and cared for.

Justice: The Highest Expression of Empathy

It's through our human connection that we discover our own humanity. Justice comes in understanding that everyone is on their own journey and has their own life purpose to answer for. When you take into account the fact that each person has their own Source light, it's easier to treat them as equals.

Empathy is thanking the hardworking cashier at the store who's slow at cashing you out because they've been on their feet for hours. It's sitting down with your four-year-old who's screaming for no reason and helping them regulate even though you're exhausted. It's looking into the eyes of someone from a different background and seeing their Soul.

Justice means you can honor your anxiety about someone and still make space for their humanity. Justice also takes knowing when you're not employing the best listening skills and correcting course. It takes consciously changing your patterns that harm others and apologizing when you've been hurtful. When you heal your pain, you stop lashing out. This ends the ripple effect of disconnection. You can then contribute to the collective healing.

Honoring another takes intention and commitment. Do you remember a moment when someone did or said something that influenced your life for the better? When you extend a kindness, you're staying connected to the web that unifies all Souls.

Sympathy: Lowest Expression of Empathy

When you feel sympathy for someone, you feel sorry for them. That's a power-over situation. Taking pity on someone puts you into the drama triangle where you play out the rescuer role to someone else's victimhood.[106] Once on that triangle, you can fall into the role of persecutor as well.

Sympathy is rescuing. Rescuing looks like doing someone's homework for them, giving someone a job when that person has no interest in working, or doing chores for someone because they won't. Sympathy is control. When you act from a rescuer position, you are stealing someone else's power to make choices for themselves.

You are responsible for your own journey. When we make a positive difference in someone's life, you are meeting them where they're at, honoring their struggle without fixing it.

To create positive engagement, slow down and listen. This is ventral vagal engagement for both parties. Genuinely hearing allows someone to calm. Meeting someone where they are at and not expecting them to have the same outlook as you is truly making a difference.

---

106. Karpman, "Karpman's Triangle."

EXERCISE
Violet Flame Visualization

I briefly mentioned Saint Germain and the violet flame at the beginning of this chapter. He is considered an "ascended master." The violet flame visualization releases all that no longer serves you. It's a flame of mercy and healing that does not burn but transforms. The image of the violet flame helps to transmute denser, old energies you may be carrying around.

This meditation cleanses the energy in both your body and etheric fields. I find it to be quite powerful. Here is one way to do it:

- Sit or lay down.
- Relax and pull your breaths all the way down into your legs, releasing tension. Breathe into your torso, and soften your stomach.
- Imagine a ball of violet flame above your head. Sit for a moment, and join with the energy.
- Once you feel the connection, let the violet flame drop down over your head. Ask the flame to cleanse all energies that no longer serve you.
- See the radiant flame stream down around your neck and shoulders. Invite the warmth in.
- Breathe deep. Pull the violet flame into your nostrils, throat, and ears. Draw the energy down into your chest, heart, and diaphragm with another deep breath.
- Continue to ask the flame to release old hurts or connections that no longer serve you.

- Trusting the energy of the flame, allow it to comb through areas of your body that need alignment. Give it the time it needs to do the cleansing.
- Speak this invocation:

Flame of mercy. Flame of forgiveness.
Thank you for your healing transformation.

Sit for a while and see how you feel following this visualization. When I use this exercise, there are times I bring the flame up from the ground and into my legs and root chakra first. Try doing it this way during another meditation. Examine how the energy feels and how this works for you.

Reality Is Relative

My reality is different from yours. My reality comes to me based upon a tapestry of events in my life and how I choose to interpret them. So does yours. When we can honor this concept, we can honor those around us.

When you create the illusion that yours is the "right" reality, then you choose to remain stoic and separate from those who have the possibility to enrich your life. Far too many times people attempt to enforce their reality on others. You can see this play out in the world, and it always has. Personally, I see this a lot in the couples work I do.[107]

Often, neither partner takes the time to ask the other's perspective. Both feel directly threatened if their loved one sees a situation differently. Honoring another's perspective does not mean you lose yours. Consider the discussion on emotional boundaries

---

107. Hendrix and Hunt, *Getting the Love You Want,* 34.

we had in chapter 5. There's a difference between trying to understand another and absorbing their opinion as your own.

It is in the space between each other that honest connection lies because that space is in constant negotiation. When we make room for another's perspective without absorbing what they think, feel, or say, we can be present to their reality in a calm way. This not only applies to our loved ones but everyone around us. This is empathy at work.

Knowing your reality is the key to having good inner boundaries. This makes operating from the dimensions of empathy much easier. Through grace, we can be present to someone else.

Jaron's Story: When Being Right Is Wrong

Jaron was a thirty-year-old male who came into therapy because he was about to lose his job. His second girlfriend in a year had just left him. Jaron spent the first session complaining that neither girlfriend "got it" and how the department head he worked for was stupid. He didn't reveal right away that he had also thrown a chair across the room during a heated debate in a meeting. Once he did, we discussed how he was lucky not to have been arrested.

Each time he came to session, he complained about the idiotic servers at the restaurants he had been in, the stupid drivers on the road, or anyone else he perceived as someone who slowed him down or got in his way. Getting Jaron to focus on emotions other than self-righteous outrage was an effort. His battle with the world was really a battle with himself turned outward.

Jaron's breakthrough came when his mother left his father. She told Jaron she had grown weary of the fighting and constantly having to defend herself from her husband. Jaron seemed shocked by this. When we broke down why he was so upset, he was able to see how he was following along with some angry family patterns and that this scared him.

"She says he never listened to her." He shrugged, but his face was turning red. "He did call her stupid a lot."

"How did that feel to hear your father call your mother stupid all the time?"

"Well, sometimes I would have to agree." His old bravado reappeared for a moment but quickly faded. His shoulders dropped. "I feel kinda bad for her. She seems beaten down by him. She's depressed, and I'm worried about her."

"Have you ever called her stupid yourself?"

"Yes."

Jaron began to tear up. Through affirming he loved and worried about his mother, we were able to start making progress on his struggles with empathy. That day, Jaron softened enough to access true emotion.

Over the next few months, we worked through ways he could take responsibility for how he treated people. We reflected on how people may have felt during his verbal tirades. He was able to access more vulnerable emotions when we discussed times people had treated him poorly. While he struggled with his defensive strategies in some moments, he began to accept that his actions were attempts to protect his own disowned pain. He soon understood that as he was avoiding pain, he was spreading it.

Jaron started dating someone new after several months in therapy. We worked on more effective communication strategies and empathy tools. He consciously stayed present when his girlfriend was upset or needed to express difficult emotions. We worked somatically when he noticed he felt threatened by someone else's opinion, so he could access the more vulnerable emotions he was trying to cover up.

A year later, Jaron was engaged. He still worked at his old job but had been communicating with coworkers in more effective ways. Now, he comes to me to do work for what he calls his "monthly tune-up" and states he is enjoying life much better now that he doesn't lead with his rage.

Empathy Is Nonjudgement

Suspending judgment. What does this look like? When is the last time you did this?

Certainly, you can remember the last time you passed judgment. Was it this morning? Two minutes ago? Was it about something your neighbor was wearing, something that was said on your local news, or was it the thought you had about the driver next to you on your way to work?

Judgment keeps you disconnected. The separation is not just from others. It splits you from your authentic Self. Like Jaron, it pushes back against feeling perceived vulnerabilities. When you fear feeling, you cultivate protective strategies—such as judgment—that hurt others.

The aggressive output that judgment requires keeps us on the offense. Sometimes, they are covert acts, and sometimes, they're overt acts. Sometimes, they are quick thoughts, and sometimes, they are full-on character assaults.

When we judge, we have to make up a narrative that allows us to stay bubbled up in our own version of what life should be. We no longer have to care about someone or even consider the world from their point of view. We can stay comforted in our little nest of superiority.

Empathy is the intention to suspend judgment. There is emotional mastery with empathy because it requires consistency. It is true skillfulness.

EXERCISE
Empathy Visualization

The best way to shift or obtain anything is to first see it in our mind's eye. Try this visualization, which applies third eye chakra activation with crown chakra energy.

- Think of a person you struggle to get along with.
- Imagine that person standing across from you.
- Take time to look at that person. Look into their face, and see what's in their eyes.
- Notice how you feel as you do this. Are you threatened? Take that deeper. Are you scared? Angry? Lonely? Rejected? Hurt? Sad?
- Now look around and to both sides of this person. What's behind them? What's to the sides of that person?
- Are there artifacts? Images? People?
- What do the images beside them tell you about how they have learned to manage their world?
- What are you understanding about them now that you see what they are dealing with?
- What emotions and thoughts are coming up for you now?
- What pains in their own being do they mirror in you?

Write down what is being mirrored. What are you noticing by journaling these answers? How are you feeling about these answers? The above visualization is ongoing and deep in its effects. Continue to journal and process this throughout the coming days and weeks as this is transformative, sometimes complex work.

EXERCISE
Writing Prompt: Empathy Reflection

Reflecting on our past injuries to others can be embarrassing, but we have all taken part in those moments. Whether it was on the elementary school playground or in the work boardroom, we have all acted out in defense of something in us at the expense of another.

Using your journal and the following prompts, write about a time you've hurt someone and explore what you would change or how you would like to make amends.

- If you got to go back in time to a moment when you said or did something that hurt someone, what would you do or say differently now?
- How can you apologize to that individual in your own writing now?
- Can you apply the Hawaiian prayer of forgiveness from chapter 8 in your journaling?

Summary

The crown chakra leads you upward into the realm of the Divine. Through this chakra, you draw energy into your system to recharge and transform. When you're open to it, the crown chakra fuels your system with light, safety, and a connection to the greater collective.

The crown chakra sits at the center of your skull and resides between the prefrontal lobe and the parietal lobe of your brain. The left and right branches of the vagus nerve start here, in cranial nerve X, and traverse down your body, connecting their branches to your organs and other systems that generate messages of safety.

The energy in this chakra is the dimension of empathy. When we can apply empathy by reflecting what people mirror in us, we can facilitate healing in ourselves and those around us.

PART 3
DEEPENING YOUR WORK

CHAPTER 11
THE SPIRITUALITY OF HEALING FROM TRAUMA

———•———

Strength does not always mean "enduring." Living with trauma is not a marathon with the gold going to the person who runs the farthest and hardest while in pain.

An archaic misconception about managing trauma is that if you cannot "handle it," you're weak. Given what you have learned thus far about how your brain and nervous system process information and conditions of safety, you can understand that responses to trauma have nothing to do with character flaws. What appears to be emotional or social skills deficits are adapted physiological reactions that play themselves out when we engage with others.

The "suck it up" or "shake it off" principle doesn't apply here. Perhaps "work it through" might be a better turn of phrase. If you or someone you know has suffered a threatening event, working through it shortly afterward will help alleviate more intense reactions later. This may include talking it out with a friend, body movements, such as walking or running, breathing, bilateral stimulation, or stretching.

When a disturbing event happens, it takes your brain and central nervous system a while to catch up with the reality of what has occurred. If you "stuff down" your reaction to it with drugs or alcohol or by denying the impact—or if you dissociated because the moment was too frightening—the meaning will continue to process in your system and will eventually ask to be "heard."[108] My client Janelle experienced this when she had an inexplicable reaction to the smell of a man's aftershave.

Janelle's Story

Janelle is a happily married forty-five-year-old mother of twin, teenage daughters. She came to my office for the first time after she had collapsed and started shaking while on an outing in a park with her girlfriends.

She had been walking along the track when a man jogged by their group. As he passed, she smelled his aftershave. This triggered a memory she didn't know she had. When she was in college and out at a campus pub one night, someone spiked her drink. The next morning, she woke up alone and fully clothed on a couch in a strange apartment. She was not bruised, and her body didn't feel harmed in anyway. Janelle chalked the experience up to excessive drinking and passing out at someone's place. She assumed the person let her sleep it off on their couch.

The smell of the aftershave from the jogger in the park released a decades-old suppressed (implicit) memory from her system. Suddenly, she was able to recall a man lying on top of her. The scent of his aftershave had been so strong she would gag remembering it. More detailed (explicit) memories returned after that day in the park. She was now struggling to cope. Nightmares were keeping her awake. She was terrified every time one of her daughters left the house. She was dissociating, short-tempered, and irritable. Janelle no longer wanted to be around people and wasn't responding to her

---

108. Ogden, Minton, and Pain, *Trauma and the Body*, 38.

friend's texts. In an effort to calm herself down, she even tried to convince herself she was making the memories up.

We targeted the foggy images she was recalling using EMDR. We were able to process out the reactions her system was having over the course of a few months. The discussion of whether or not the event happened was extensive between us. She didn't want to falsely accuse someone of something that might have been consensual, albeit drunken, sex. The conversation in this case wasn't about punitive, legal measures. The two of us talked about the interpretation of the event and the meaning her body and psyche had made (that she was powerless and unsafe). We worked with how this was expressing itself in her system so she could feel clear and nonreactive and able to read situations for what they are. Janelle can now notice when she has any "residual" responses verses understanding and emotions around the event.

Our Senses Hold Memories

The first several weeks following a traumatic event is called the acute phase, according to the *DSM-5*, which is the reference manual mental health clinicians use to diagnose.[109] Managing your system during this time can help avoid more severe, defensive reactions later.

Everyone is unique. Some nervous systems are more resilient to a distressing or shocking event than others. People internalize and make meaning of situations differently. Just think of an event (traumatic or not) from childhood that your sibling has a completely different perspective of—or that they don't hold the memory of at all.

---

109. *Diagnostic of Statistical Manual of Mental Disorders*, 271.

How safe you felt with your childhood experiences and how frequently activated your sympathetic nervous system was as you grew up affects your personal dynamics later in life. I have personally found mine to be less resilient as I age. Childhood stressors—along with your garden variety life events—have me working regularly with my system. This not only includes Eye Movement Desensitization and Reprocessing (EMDR), Internal Family Systems (IFS) therapy, and regular meditation, but energy work and a healthy lifestyle as well. Engaging intentionally and in loving, healthy ways with those in my life offers me an opportunity for co-regulation. I see the management of my central nervous system as an emotional, mental, and spiritual one.

Lack of resiliency in your nervous system is not a character flaw. It's biology as it presents in your emotional, psychological, and spiritual encounters with the world. The first thing I encourage is for you to be accepting of yourself in all your complexity. The more awareness you have, the more self-care skills you can incorporate into your life. You were not responsible for your early childhood pain. You are, however, responsible for your own healing and claiming responsibility for your actions if you are perpetuating hurt onto others.

Refusing to heal brings more pain to your system than the momentary discomfort of revisiting old issues in therapy sessions to relieve them.[110] I liken the avoidance of therapeutic healing to a backpack that never gets cleaned out. It just gets heavier and bulkier through the years.

Over the last several decades, research and access to knowledge of how to heal has burgeoned. You have the gold medal at your fingertips, and you no longer have to run a marathon with

---

110. Menakem, *My Grandmother's Hands*, 19.

broken bones to get it. What healing from trauma does is free up the "false readings" in your system. Alleviating trauma responses creates space to be present to what is happening in your life as your vagus nerve and other aspects of your system, such as your chakras, can accurately calculate a situation. Trauma therapy assists you in being able to breathe again. It hands you back your Soul Self where your joy, curiosity, and genuineness already are. Psychological healing is the spiritual path.

Chakras and Trauma

In earlier chapters, I talked about how I break down the chakras into two categories—essential chakras and evolving chakras—as I work with clients. I have developed the two terms based on how I see these energy centers presenting during trauma processing. Essential chakras, root (body), sacral (emotion), and solar plexus (mind), hold the identities of the human self and the memories of early events within them. They are the energy centers that keep us pursuing biological and social needs. The evolving chakras, heart (compassion), throat (connection), third eye (spirituality), and crown (empathy), possess potential for new meaning and the ability to authentically connect with others and the Soul Self.

While I see the essential chakras rooted in past foundations and the evolving chakras as surging toward the future you, all these energy centers engage in a collective process of informing the system of both the past and present encounters. We cannot bypass to the evolving chakras if we have not healed, grounded, and restored the archaic energies hiding out in the essentials. The pain of loss can be felt just as deeply in the heart chakra as it can in the sacral. These chakras, like our biological system, cannot work independently of each other, at least not for long.

Our essential chakras are where the "children" hide out. These are the young parts of your psyche that hold experiences of attachment with your caretakers. If the early experiences were safe and loving, the energies here are balanced. However, no one gets away with a perfect childhood. The most well-meaning of parents slip up occasionally, and early childhood caretakers can make mistakes. Even if for brief moments, a child's needs might go unmet. To that infant or toddler, that moment may register as intolerable and scary. Those times of lack of safety register in the essential chakras as these were the energy centers that first came online in our human development.[111] These children are not easily beguiled into coming forth to release their convictions that the world is not a safe place for them.

Trauma Terms

Having definitions to identify your experiences empowers you to understand what is occurring. It also allows you to know when to seek help. *Trauma* is a general term that refers to the physical and emotional impact of a stressful event. Trauma is a rupture in your sense of safety and connection. When I break down the concept of trauma to my clients, I tell them that trauma is the past controlling the present and determining future outcomes.

Post-traumatic stress disorder (PTSD) describes the behaviors and outcomes to a death, threat, or serious violence.[112] PTSD and acute trauma are the only types of trauma that are diagnosed in the *Diagnostic of Statistical Manual of Mental Disorders-5*. PTSD generally references a horrific single event or few events, such as a shooting, rape, war, or natural disaster, and the affects it leaves

---

111. Judith, *Eastern Body, Western Mind*, 38.
112. *Diagnostic of Statistical Manual of Mental Disorders*, 271–72.

afterward. Reexperiencing these stimuli and the avoidance of pain can leave a person limited in all facets of their life.

Single event traumas are disturbing incidents that happened once. Depending on the intensity of the event, they can be referred to as a big trauma (big T), which is life-threatening, such as being robbed at gunpoint, or a little trauma (little t), which is not life-threatening but can be strongly impactful. An example of a little t may be a fender bender in the grocery store parking lot. That is a disturbing event that may force you to be aware the next time you drive through that area. A big T trauma would be a massive car collision. How you are treated by police or the hospital afterward may compound or alleviate the intensity of the experience.

Another term to describe a type of traumatic encounter would be *vicarious trauma*. If you are the one driving by that massive car accident, you are experiencing it vicariously. Many therapists, news reporters, and medical personnel can be exposed to the trauma of others. It's important if you work in a profession where you are constantly witnessing the trauma another person is experiencing to take good care.

Developmental and complex traumas are enormous components of trauma-related issues that many therapists see. If you grew up in a household that was violent, neglectful, or physically or emotionally unsafe, you have experienced developmental traumas.[113]

If relationship patterns continued to reinforce painful experiences in adulthood, these "realities" of a lack of safety are reinforced in your system. An abusive relationship is an example of a complex trauma.[114]

---

113. Paulsen, *Looking through the Eyes of Trauma and Dissociation*, 27.
114. Courtois and Ford, *Treating Complex Traumatic Stress Disorders*, 13.

These experiences form how you interact with others, how you manage your emotions, and how you cope with stressors as an adult. These difficult situations impede your ability to focus and slow other executive functioning abilities. You may have missed important developmental milestones as you were spending most of your time surviving. More than likely, you will grapple with dissociation (dorsal vagal responses) or an overcharged sympathetic nervous system.[115] As you have read, a lack of safety has been sending a punch to your system for years.

Sometimes, a stored traumatic event can come from medical experiences, which can be compounded if they happened when you were young. You could have had all the safe, loving connection in the world from your caretakers, but if you were forced to be still during a medical procedure or put under during a surgery and experienced pain afterward, the effects of this can be locked in your body and resurface years later.

Health issues can create trauma struggles. Our world came out of a major pandemic, which has left people with lifelong symptoms from the COVID-19 virus. People lost loved ones, and many people responded to this unsafe experience in painful ways. How children were affected by this epidemic will reveal itself over time.

Adverse childhood experiences can be assessed and worked through. If you believe you struggle with the effects of traumatic events, it's important to talk to a licensed mental health professional. This person can give you insight and information, normalize your response, and provide assessments that start the healing therapeutic process. You can form an alliance and a plan, as this person holds safe space for you.

---

115. Dana, *The Polyvagal Theory in Therapy*, 214.

Working toward a resolution of trauma doesn't require revisiting the story in ways that retraumatize you. In fact, that is a primary understanding with trauma-informed, licensed therapists. Separating autonomic responses from the old version of the story can be worked out utilizing therapeutic modalities that help stabilize your central nervous system.

Implicit Memory

Some of those "false readings" that register in your body come from times when you have no memory of being hurt. That is called an implicit memory. Implicit memory is when you hold emotional intensity in your body, but your brain can't attach a situation to logical memory. This generally happens when we are young, before parts of your brain were able to register events explicitly.[116] It can also happen to someone who is rendered unconscious due to drugs or alcohol.

The responses to these memories flare up in your system and feel like fear, longing, or anger. That confuses the conscious mind and can bring on a level of distrust about emotions because the physiological responses feel nebulous. The reason they are so intense is because as a child, feeling is all you had. You didn't have a voice or a logical thought process by which to communicate. You certainly had limited means to protect yourself. As a child, you simply felt the fears.

When you have an experience like this, it can help to tell yourself this is an "implicit response." Being able to breathe through them and identify where you feel them in your body is a wonderful way to map and heal them with your therapist. An infant holds only implicit memory. They don't have the brain development for language, higher reasoning, or to physically provide for their

---

116. Lanius, Paulsen, and Corrigan, *Neurobiology and Treatment of Traumatic Dissociation*, 208.

needs, but never *ever* think they don't feel what is occurring around them. Those experiences are stored in their system and are felt.

Explicit Memory

Explicit memory is when you can tell a story about what happened. You may have chronological order or images and can apply logic and meaning. When you think of memory, you generally think it looks like an explicit one. This part of our brain comes online around three years old, and logic begins to refine itself around five.

All memory is biased. We make meaning of situations based on our reality and how the situations impacted us. The mental health community used to believe that talking about trauma was the best approach. If a client was able to recount incidences without any emotions, it was generally thought that they were healed. Decades of research has shown us a different way.[117]

Talking without emotion could mean you have developed strategies of disconnection to manage overwhelming physiological responses. It's another form of dissociation. It's the opposite of living toward an embodiment of yourself.

EXERCISE
Four-Way Breathing

This is another technique to continue with grounding through breath. As I mentioned, one way to engage and calm through connection of the ventral vagal nerve is slower breathing, particularly on the exhale. This exercise also opens the energy of the heart chakra.

---

117. Lanius, Paulsen, and Corrigan, *Neurobiology and Treatment of Traumatic Dissociation*, 220.

- Bring in a breath and slowly count to four on the in breath.
- Hold the breath deep in your lungs for four more slow counts.
- Exhale for four slow counts.
- Then hold the breath for four slow counts before repeating the cycle.

As you repeat, notice the energy in your body. Has it expanded in your chest? Is your heart rate slower? What is the overall feeling in your body? How do you feel emotionally?

Avoidance of Pain Is Avoidance of a Life Well Lived

Traumatic responses may show up in less obvious ways such as constant agitation, aggressive behaviors, victimized thinking that blames others, poor sleep and sleep hygiene, a short or explosive temper, over- or undereating, obsessive thinking, or an inability to be present to yours or another's complicated emotions. Dissociation might look more subtle and doesn't always show itself on a higher, more obvious spectrum.

When you don't listen to those aspects of yourself that are asking to be healed, your system will become chronically anxious and/or depressed. You either attempt to control everything or avoid everything that you can't control. Life becomes a chronic thrumming of discontent, so you reach for things outside of you to escape. This is the root of addictive patterns.[118]

Numbing with various sources keeps you from feeling. Reaching for stimulating things creates the illusion of fabulousness. When you think of addictive behaviors, you think mostly of an abuse or

---

118. Nakken, *The Addictive Personality*, 35.

dependence on drugs or alcohol, but anything outside of you that is constantly pursued to alter your mood is addictive. Maladaptive ways of soothing keep you from fully being present. Reality doesn't have to be bleak and intense. Life is not always full of pain unless you continue to let it be.

Trauma Released

To describe what it feels like once you have worked through issues related to trauma requires a lot of adjectives. Here are a few: *light, free, clear, open, peaceful, joyful, grounded, secure, safe, serene,* and *playful.*

Clients have reported they can breathe deeply again. Some report they are able to have access to actual emotion and not an intense physiological response that locked them down for years. Others have said they can think about their past without intensity in their body—or even without fearing the possibility of that intensity. Others say they can just think, without a foggy brain. Trauma clearing alleviates rapid anger issues, general crankiness, poor sleep patterns, and—potentially—nightmares.

Freeing up these "punches," as I refer to them with clients, lays the groundwork for new pathways in your life. Like having used a machete to clear brush, your view of the world is suddenly clearer. Your light shines brighter. You circle back to that childlike essence inside of you—that energy you forgot about. It's the warmth of coming home in safe, happy ways.

Resourcing

Resourcing refers to shoring up your system with caring, grounding, and calming approaches. These might include ways to identify and learn how to reengage with your system because you have coped with stressors in the past by dissociating through dorsal vagal shut down. They may be ways that help you calm your sympathetic responses.

Resourcing, simply put, is offering resources for you. They are applied methods that teach you how to manage your emotional responses when you struggle or cope with the feelings presenting in your body. Resourcing could even look like mapping out boundaries with others to help you feel that you have more psychological room to get to know yourself. Many of the exercises in this book are resources for you to access. They are intended to help you feel safer, feel more grounded, and engage in innovative ways with your world.

Revisit the chapters on the chakras and how they connect to the vagus nerve, including some of the writing prompts and boundary scripts. Notice the ones that feel the safest for you. As you work through some, you may find you can do others that were not comfortable for you in the beginning. Go slow through them. The intention is to get you to befriend your body and ultimately find safety within it.

A trauma therapist will work with you on what I refer to as "resourcing." Each client responds differently to various techniques. Some techniques may be:

- Safety messaging, such as utilizing the five senses for grounding.
- Getting you accustomed to your body with walking or stretching.
- Calming techniques with tapping, bilateral stimulation with supportive visualizations, or meditation.
- Creativity with visualization, drawing, mapping, or sound therapy.

Therapists help you restore your system and help you apply these skills. These are just some of the ways to replenish your psyche and bring joy back into your mind and body. When you have more adaptable ways to manage intensity in your system, it is easy to process old memories.

EXERCISE
Writing Prompt: Time for Deeper Reflection

How are you feeling about yourself now that you understand your body holds the information you need to heal? Let's do some reflecting on what some of your self-soothing strategies are. Are they hurting you or bringing you joy? Write out the answers to these questions in your journal.

- What are ways you relax after a long day?
- Do you think they help? Are the effects long term or short term?
- How do you feel about those relaxation techniques? Check in with your body on this.
- What emotions come up as a result of thinking about your self-soothing strategies? Calm, happy, or sadness? Worry or shame?
- If these are techniques you feel hurt you in the long run, do a reverse emotional check and ask yourself what emotions come up first before you employ those techniques.
- Where do you feel them in your body? What are they telling you?

Summary

When you continue to "suck it up" and run from emotional discomfort, you exhaust yourself on all levels. That is when you reach for self-soothing techniques outside of yourself that are maladaptive to avoid emotional and physiological pain. While you didn't cause your childhood pain, it is yours to work through and heal.

PTSD usually refers to single events of trauma. Big T traumas are another reference to life-threatening traumas. Little t's are traumas that may not be life-threatening but affect you deeply. Both big T traumas and little t traumas can be single events or occur regularly. When unsafe occurrences are regular or have happened multiple times, you have experienced complex trauma.

If you grew up in a household that was constantly unsafe, your developmental process, which is generally referred to as developmental trauma, was hindered. You may hold various traumatic experiences in your system that reveal themselves through depression or anxiety. Some childhood memories could be explicit, which are chronological in nature and have words or places to help describe an event. Some memories are implicit and are stored in the body. Implicit memories occur because your brain was too young to remember chronological details, or you may have been dissociated.

Trauma is stored in your central nervous system and brain. Trauma reveals itself in multiple ways that are not always extreme or obvious in nature. These experiences can be general malaise, irritability, avoidance of conflict, or desire to control. A trauma-informed therapist will help you work through stored responses and miscues in your central nervous system.

CHAPTER 12
SOOTHING AND ENGAGING THE VAGUS NERVE AND CHAKRAS

H ave you ever fully checked your posture? Perhaps you've passed yourself in a window on the street or caught sight of yourself in a full-length mirror when you were focused on other things beside your image. What did you notice? How do you hold your body during everyday movements? Do you struggle with moving, or do you struggle with resting? Where do you feel over-worked in your body when you walk? Do you walk much?

While I am not a physical therapist, I can generally gauge some-one's overall emotional well-being based on how they carry them-selves. An anxious, hypervigilant person will sit more erect with shoulders tight. Hands may be clenched or firmly set, as if on the ready to be used. They may have a hard time sitting still in a chair without distractions. Eyes might be wider because of a need to keep watch. All this is stimulating fight or flight responses from the sym-pathetic regions of the vagus nerve.

On the other hand, a depressed person will generally slump in a protective, forward posture that disconnects them from the chakras and most of the vagus nerve. Their back and ribs are more exposed in an effort to shield their softer, more vulnerable front from pain. This pulls in and down on the internal organs, which disengages the ventral or sympathetic system and activates the dorsal vagal nerve of disconnection.

Muscle tone can be an indicator of how connected someone is to their body and their surroundings as well. A body that moves will have more taut muscles because the individual is using them more frequently. A person who is disconnected from their body and not moving much will have less tone and perhaps more body fat, as eating may be the choice of grounding and comfort. Too much weight on our bodies can be an armor intended to keep people from getting close. Too much food can be an effort to calm the system into a dorsal vagal response and emotionally soothe.

None of this is intended to shame the reader. This is not a discussion about perfect body composition or obtaining it. Our physical form is simply a rapid indicator of how we interact with our world. Even animals carry themselves based on their interpretations of life experiences. It's simply a very mammalian response.

Our bodies are the sentinel to our inner well-being. This chapter is intended to provide more insight and opportunities to connect with it. Try out some of the movements in the following exercise and notice how you feel.

EXERCISE
Move Differently

For this exercise, you will have to put your book down, so read what I have written before you do. This is a very simple process. Just move.

- Stand up and move in ways you are not familiar with. Reach your arms up to the sky and hold. Lift your legs like you are marching or high kicking (if it's safe).

Stretch your neck, torso, or lower back. Make sure the movements are different than you are used to.

- As you shift from one stretch to another, hold and count to twenty. This gives your muscles enough time to code the memory into your body and get a good stretch.

- Enjoy the newness of the experience and notice how you feel emotionally.

Lois's Story: How Our Bodies Respond to a Lack of Safety—Whether We Like It or Not

Lois had been in a psychologically, emotionally, and financially abusive relationship for two decades. She had made it clear to me as we began our work years earlier that she wasn't going to leave the marriage until her three children were in college. She also stated the reason she chose to stay for now was that her husband was never home because he traveled for work. She believed that with him gone so often, she could do right by the children without them observing too much abuse.

"They could stay in their school system and have some means until they get out of college. Then I can find a full-time job and support myself," she told me when we started. "Besides, he's not hitting me. Except," her voice dropped, "with his words."

As hard as it was for me to watch her being treated so poorly, I agreed to take her on as a client. Our agreement was that she would have to leave the house with the children and have an emergency escape plan if the husband got physically abusive, as I also had a duty to warn the authorities if they were unsafe. She agreed.

Her therapeutic goal with me was to understand how she had "picked" someone like this as her spouse to begin with. She knew he was with other women and that he might have been seeking anonymous sex when he was on the road. Porn was all over his computer and phone. When she did finally leave, she would tell me, she didn't want to repeat the same relationship patterns later on. In effect, Lois was choosing to stay in the eye of the storm until the rest of her family was out and she had a handle on what went wrong to begin with.

Lois lived a physically healthy lifestyle but suffered from extreme fatigue, back pain, and inflammation.

"I work out constantly, run, swim—I'm at the gym four days a week," she said. "I watch what I eat, yet I'm thirty pounds heavier than what my doctor says is healthy for someone as short as I am."

We agreed not to discuss weight or body image in any way, as this was also her husband's favorite verbally abusive tactic to get her to feel bad. We spent our time understanding abuse cycles and how they played out in her childhood home as well as her marriage. She started to understand addiction isn't always drug related. She learned healthy boundaries and what enabling other's addictive behaviors looked like.

One day, she came into our session and said, "I've talked to an attorney and filed for divorce."

Her children were in early middle school, not college the way her exit strategy had been.

"I can't stay anymore." She shrugged. "I have more power than I thought I had. I can't live like this."

In the years following her divorce, Lois physically changed. She had stepped into her own emotional well-being and was now safe in her own home. She no longer struggled with inflammation and her back pain was gone.

"I've lost twenty-five pounds," she said. "Even though I know I'm not supposed to talk about it. I haven't done anything differently. It just started to pour off of me this past year."

"Funny what stress will do to your body, isn't it?" I said.

"That's a fact," she said. "I feel so good. I wish I had understood how my body hurt back then because I felt like I was in a constant war zone."

Our Spine Holds Up More Than Our Body

The spine. It's the metaphorical motherboard of your physical and intuitive processing system. Your central nervous system, brain, and etherical energies do some constant, deep work with the help of the spine. Unlike some body parts, you cannot live without your spine.

Enlivening your torso, engaging through yoga, doing Pilates, stretching, and breathing supports your sense of grounding and helps you decipher messages from the inside out.[119] It's that internal locus of control that develops your understanding of how the world works. It starts with the spine and how healthy it is.

Yogis have understood for centuries that flexibility of the spine alleviates physical as well as emotional aging. Being properly grounded to the earth isn't a dense sensation of immobility. Being ungrounded to the earth creates an inability to connect to yourself as well as others. Neither of these moves you along. The aging process is not just physical. It's cognitive as well. Why rush it with a lack of self-care?

---

119. Ogden and Fisher, *Sensorimotor Psychotherapy*, 356.

EXERCISE
Waking Up the Spine

This exercise is best if you have secure footing, perhaps with sneakers. It is intended to engage the muscles in your legs, which open the root chakra and chakras in the feet for grounding. The arms are slipped behind your back to bring on full engagement of the ventral vagal energy—all the chakras and spinal cord.

Your head is lightly tilted as well, which frees up energy in your heart, throat, third eye, and crown chakras, which are deeply connected to ventral vagal wellness.

- Square your feet to the ground and find your secure footing.
- Slip your arms around your back.
- Squat to a level that is not aggressive but helps to engage the thigh muscles.
- Tilt your head back.
- Draw in a breath and slowly exhale.
- Slowly stand straight again and notice how your body feels.

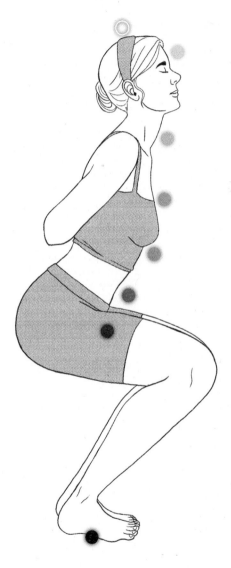

Figure 6: Vagus Stretch

Connecting

Connection has a flexibility to it. There's energy in the earth and the sky. Engaging in the energy of the spine is necessary to thrive. Open up your hands and embrace a tree. Take your shoes off and feel the grass. Turn your face to the sky and feel the light. Let your heart be part of this process. Breathe. Use the power of your autonomic senses to pull air deeper into your body to soothe your system. Here is a great exercise for that.

EXERCISE
Breathing from the Heart

This exercise is intended to engage ventral vagal activity and open the throat and heart chakras. Stand as you do this to incorporate your body and get the full benefit of the breath. Hold onto the back of a chair or secure your hands on a counter if necessary. Do not tilt your head backward of forward; just keep it straight.

- Turn your head to left and wait until you yawn.
- Slowly return your head to a straight facing position.
- Turn your head to right and wait until you yawn.
- How do you feel?

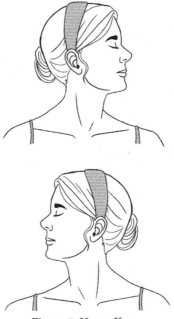

Figure 7: Vagus Yawn

Summary

This chapter was intended to give you further exercises as a way to prepare for deeper trauma processing with a therapist. Grounding and safety are paramount to a healthy system.

Some of these exercises may help you understand how you manage your system when you're not even thinking about it. If we're anxious in posture and ready for a fight, then we are too constricted to tune in. We have no access to our chakric energy and are overengaging the sympathetic nerve. The same happens if we have shut off the front portions of our body by slumping, as the energies get closed off in an effort to protect.

As always, I encourage you to reach beyond a comfort limit without pushing yourself into a state where you want to shut down. When we grow, we stretch. However, we have to understand where our window of tolerance is. This way we can create the space to absorb new information. Healing is growth, and growth has an exponential quality to it. Find your emotional pace by being present to your body.

CONCLUSION

———•———

I t took years of watching my clients' somatic processing to understand the strong correlation between their vagus nerve and their chakras and how these messaging centers overlapped. It took just as long before I considered putting what I observed into the public forum. After all, I'm a clinician. How would this information be received? What would my colleagues think of me? However, if we are honest, most clinicians see the inexplicable energetic shifts that occur while we work in service of others. So, let's take this discussion out of the box and apply it when it helps. Let's take the etheric and put it into the licensed mental health clinician's room to pull from when needed.

My profession has developed this past hundred years from a belief in a white, male-driven psychosexual model to behavior and thought theories to now (and thankfully) understanding our body absorbs and processes life information in multiple ways. As we seek to help people facilitate healthy approaches in relationships with others and themselves, I can't help but to rejoice in the rapidity and elevation of this growth.

There are far too many qualities to our human condition that cannot be—and probably will never be—measured. Trusting in the intuitive engagement is just part of the collaborative experience. I hope that you, too, will trust your own intuition in becoming whole again. Lean into your soft spots. Remember that discomfort is information just asking to be heard.

The individual choices you make ripple outward and influence those around you. For every person you affect, many more absorb the result of your actions or words. We are a collective whether we like it or not. If you never fully understand how the chakras and vagus nerve engage energetically, I hope this book has helped you to ask deeper questions about your personal history and what you may need to heal. The healing of old wounds helps to shift the small circles around you. Those circles then shift and so on.

Once you know something, you can't go back to pretending you don't. Allow for expansion and know that, at times, it can be messy and uncertain. Commit to being present so you can heal the past. I wish you all the caring and safety you need. Find your peace.

Thank you.

ACKNOWLEDGMENTS

•————————•

My heartfelt gratitude to Andrea McCabe, MS, who sat through countless hours, years, rewrites, and cheerleading calls; Ann Clark, PhD, my friend, Reiki Master, and fellow brainstormer; trauma therapist, Chris Causey, MA, MDiv, a man of great insight and support personally and professionally; Celeste Bradley, who's buoyed me through years of writing escapades; Charlie Fitch, who can rock a branding; Dr. Peter Jezewski, for the lending of his precious anatomy books and notes; and my son, who watched over me through the deadline process and beyond.

Thank you to my acquisitions editor, Angela Wix, for "getting it" and guiding me through the book doula process and to the wonderful staff at Llewellyn Publishing who have steered this manuscript into its current, beautiful form.

I am forever moved and grateful to all my clients who have entrusted me to travel alongside them during their healing journeys. To the readers who are looking for peace in this sometimes muddled world. Healing is forever at hand if you seek it.

RECOMMENDED RESOURCES

———•———

B elow is a list of reading and resources that will help you get started on your journey of becoming trauma informed. As you read, notice how the information is affecting you. If you become overly stimulated, agitated, worried, or out of sorts in any way, this may be an indicator that the reading is stimulating unresolved traumatic issues. On the other hand, this information is also empowering as it may provide you with some definitions and descriptions that were indecipherable before. Your system will lead the way as the body is its own communication messenger and needs to be trusted. Stay attuned to yourself as you read.

These books are designed for mainstream reading and are not textbooks. They are accessible, supportive to the process of raising awareness, and well-informed by people who work in the trauma field. This reading list can lead you to other forms of helpful information.

If you are looking for a therapist, ask someone who is already working with one. A master's level or PhD licensed therapist will be the level of education you are seeking.

Licensed therapists have a vast array of focuses and training. You are looking for a trauma-informed therapist with modalities that have known validity to help alleviate symptoms of trauma in your body. If you can't find anyone in your area, a list of licensed therapists can be found on Psychology Today's website. A Google search can assist you in finding someone as well. Do your research and trust your "gut." Working with a therapist is a bonding experience that takes time and requires trust. Therapists in the United States are licensed within their state of practice; however, states are developing laws of reciprocity that are allowing therapists to work with clients in other states in an online telehealth capacity.

Basic Trauma Information

The Body Keeps the Score: Brain, Mind, and Body in the Healing of Trauma by Bessel van der Kolk

In an Unspoken Voice: How the Body Releases Trauma and Restores Goodness by Peter A. Levine

My Grandmother's Hands: Racialized Trauma and the Pathway to Mending Our Hearts and Bodies by Resmaa Menakem

Waking the Tiger: Healing Trauma by Peter A. Levine

Chakras and Yoga

Eastern Body, Western Mind: Psychology and the Chakra System as a Path to the Self by Anodea Judith

Eye of the Lotus: Psychology of the Chakras by Richard Jelusich

Light on Life: The Yoga Journey to Wholeness, Inner Peace, and Ultimate Freedom by B. K. S. Iyengar

Theory of the Chakras: Bridge to Higher Consciousness by Hiroshi Motoyama

Therapeutic Yoga for Trauma Recovery: Applying the Principles of Polyvagal Theory for Self-Discovery, Embodied Healing, and Meaningful Change by Arielle Schwartz

EMDR (Eye Movement Desensitization Reprocessing)

Brainspotting: The Revolutionary New Therapy for Rapid and Effective Change by David Grand

Getting Past Your Past: Take Control of Your Life with Self-Help Techniques from EMDR Therapy by Francine Shapiro

Internal Family Systems

Internal Family Systems Therapy by Richard C. Schwartz

The Mosaic Mind: Empowering the Tormented Selves of Child Abuse Survivors by Regina A. Goulding and Richard C. Schwartz

No Bad Parts: Healing Trauma & Restoring Wholeness with the Internal Family Systems Model by Richard C. Schwartz

Grounding in Your Body

Accessing the Healing Power of the Vagus Nerve: Self-Help Exercises for Anxiety, Depression, Trauma, and Autism by Stanley Rosenberg

Anchored: How to Befriend Your Nervous System Using Polyvagal Theory by Deb Dana

Becoming Safely Embodied: A Guide to Organize Your Mind, Body, and Heart to Feel Secure in the World by Deirdre Fay

Polyvagal Exercises for Safety and Connection: 50 Client-Centered Practices by Deb Dana

Mindfulness

Buddha's Brain: The Practical Neuroscience of Happiness, Love & Wisdom by Rick Hanson

Full Catastrophe Living: Using the Wisdom of Your Body and Mind to Face Stress, Pain, and Illness by Jon Kabat-Zinn

Mindfulness in Plain English by Bhante Henepola Gunaratana

Radical Compassion: Learning to Love Yourself and Your World with the Practice of RAIN by Tara Branch

Seeking the Heart of Wisdom: The Path of Insight Meditation by Joseph Goldstein and Jack Kornfield

Training the Mind and Cultivating Loving-Kindness by Chögyam Trungpa

When Things Fall Apart: Heart Advice for Difficult Times by Pema Chödrön

Polyvagal Theory

The Pocket Guide to the Polyvagal Theory: The Transformative Power of Feeling Safe by Stephen W. Porges

Polyvagal Safety: Attachment, Communication, Self-Regulation by Stephen W. Porges

Spirituality from the Perspective of the Soul

Destiny of Souls: New Case Studies of Life Between Lives by Michael Newton

Journey of Souls: Case Studies of the Life Between Lives by Michael Newton

The Seat of the Soul by Gary Zukav

Through Time into Healing: Discovering the Power of Regression Therapy to Ease Trauma and Transform Mind, Body, and Relationships by Brian L. Weiss

Wisdom of Souls: Case Studies of Life Between Lives from the Michael Newton Institute by The Newton Institute

BIBLIOGRAPHY

Abbate, Skya. *The Hara, the Source of Life and the Navel, the Gate of Spirit*. Acupuncture College. https://acupuncturecollege.edu/blog/hara-source-life-and0navel-gate-spirit.

Alcantara, Margarita. *Chakra Healing: A Beginner's Guide to Self-Healing Techniques that Balance the Chakras*. New York: Fall River Press, 2017.

Bach, Donna, Gary Groesbeck, Peta Stapleton, Rebecca Sims, Katharina Blickheuser, and Dawson Church. "Clinical EFT (Emotional Freedom Techniques) Improves Multiple Physiological Markers of Health." *Journal of Evidence-Based Integrative Medicine* 24 (February 2019). https://doi.org/10.1177/2515690X18823691.

Brach, Tara. *Radical Compassion: Learning to Love Yourself and Your World with the Practice of RAIN*. New York: Penguin Random House, 2019.

Cannon, Dolores. *Between Death and Life: Conversations with a Spirit*. Dublin: Gill Books, 2003.

Caron, Christina. "The Vast Potential of the Vagus Nerve." *New York Times*, June 2, 2022, New York edition.

Carter, Rita, Susan Aldridge, Martyn Page, and Steve Parker. *The Human Brain Book: An Illustrated Guide to its Structure, Function, and Disorders*. New York: DK Publishing, 2014.

Courtois, Christine A., and Julian D. Ford, eds. *Treating Complex Traumatic Stress Disorders: Scientific Foundations and Therapeutic Models*. New York: The Guilford Press, 2009.

Dana, Deb. *Anchored: How to Befriend Your Nervous System Using Polyvagal Theory*. Boulder, CO: Sounds True, 2021.

———. *The Polyvagal Theory in Therapy: Engaging the Rhythm of Regulation*. New York: W. W. Norton & Company, 2018.

Diagnostic of Statistical Manual of Mental Disorders: DSM-5. Washington, DC: American Psychiatric Association, 2013.

Eden, Donna. *Energy Medicine: Balancing Your Body's Energy for Optimal Health, Joy, and Vitality*. London: Penguin Group, 2008.

Evans, Patricia. *Controlling People: How to Recognize, Understand, and Deal with People Who Try to Control You*. Avon, MA: Adams Media Corp, 2002.

Feinstein, David, Donna Eden, and Gary Craig. *The Promise of Energy Psychology: Revolutionary Tools for Dramatic Personal Change*. New York: Penguin Group, 2005.

Feucht, Andrea. "The Vagus Nerve: The Key to Unlock the Gut/Brain/and Body Connection." Innovative Medicine. https://innovativemedicine.com/the-vagus-nerve-the-key-to-unlock-the-gut-brain-and-body-connection/.

Fossella, Tina. "Human Nature, Buddha Nature: An Interview with John Welwood." Tricycle Magazine, Spring 2011. http://www.tinafossella.com/articles/2015/2/13/human-nature-buddha-nature.

Frankl, Viktor E. *Man's Search for Meaning*. Boston: Beacon Press, 2006.

"Gaslighting." *Psychology Today*. Accessed 2022. https://www.psychologytoday.com/us/basics/gaslighting.

Goenka, S.N., Sayadaw, Ledi, *Mindfulness Based Stress Reduction: Mindfulness of Breathing: Proprioception* (U Ba Khin, vipassana, Mindfulness, 11.1,194202. https://link.springer.com/article/10.1007/s12671-019-01259-8).

Goodchild, Chloe. *The Naked Voice: Transforming Your Life through the Power of Sound*. Berkeley: North Atlantic Books, 2015.

Grand, David. *Brainspotting: The Revolutionary New Therapy for Rapid and Effective Change*. Boulder, CO: Sounds True, 2013.

Hanson, Rick. *Buddha's Brain: The Practical Neuroscience of Happiness, Love & Wisdom*. Oakland, CA: New Harbinger Publications, 2009.

Hendrix, Harville, and Helen LaKelly Hunt. *Getting the Love You Want: A Guide for Couples*. New York: St. Martin's Griffin, 2019.

Iyengar, B. K. S. *Light on Yoga: The Bible of Modern Yoga—Its Philosophy and Practice—by the World's Foremost Teacher*. New York: Schocken Books, 1976.

Judith, Anodea. *Eastern Body, Western Mind: Psychology and the Chakra System as a Path to the Self*. Berkeley: Celestial Arts, 2004.

Judith, Anodea, and Lion Goodman. *Creating on Purpose: The Spiritual Technology of Manifesting through the Chakras*. Boulder, CO: Sounds True, 2012.

Judith, Anodea, and Selene Vega. *The Sevenfold Journey: Reclaiming Mind, Body & Spirit through the Chakras*. Freedom, CA: The Crossing Press, 1993.

Jung, C. G. *The Psychology of Kundalini Yoga: Notes on the Seminar Given in 1939 by C. G. Jung*. Edited by Sonu Shamdasani. Princeton: Princeton University Press, 1996.

Johari, Harish. *Chakras: Energy Centers of Transformation*. Rochester, VT: Destiny Books, 2000.

Kabat-Zinn, Jon. *Full Catastrophe Living: Using the Wisdom of Your Body and Mind to Face Stress, Pain, and Illness*. New York: Bantam Books, 2013.

Karpman, Stephen. "Karpman's Triangle." Karpman Drama Triangle. https://www.karpmandramatriangle.com.

Kawasaki, Hiroto, and Chandan G. Reddy. "Investigation of Human Cognition in Epilepsy Surgery Patients." In *Youmans Neurological Surgery*, edited by H. Richard Winn, 734–42. Philadelphia: W. B. Saunders, 2004.

Khamisa, Azim. *Azim's Bardo: From Murder to Forgiveness: A Father's Journey*. Cardiff, CA: Waterside Press, 1998.

Kunz, Dora, and Dolores Krieger. *The Spiritual Dimensions of Therapeutic Touch*. Rochester, VT: Bear & Co., 2004.

Lanius, Ulrich F., Sandra L. Paulsen, and Frank M. Corrigan, eds. *Neurobiology and Treatment of Traumatic Dissociation: Toward an Embodied Self*. New York: Springer Publishing Company, 2014.

Levine, Peter A. *Waking the Tiger: Healing Trauma: The Innate Capacity to Transform Overwhelming Experiences*. Berkeley: North Atlantic Books, 1997.

Linn, Denise. *Sacred Space: Clearing and Enhancing the Energy of Your Home*. New York: Ballantine Books, 1995.

Luft, Joe, and Harrington Ingham. "The Johari Window: A Graphic Model of Interpersonal Awareness." Proceedings of the Western Training Laboratory in Group Development. Los Angeles: UCLA, 1955.

Menakem, Resmaa. *My Grandmother's Hands: Racialized Trauma and the Pathway to Mending Our Hearts and Bodies*. Las Vegas: Central Recovery Press, 2017.

Maslow, A. H. "'Higher' and 'Lower' Needs." *The Journal of Psychology: Interdisciplinary and Applied* 25, no. 2 (1948): 433–36. https://doi.org/10.1080/00223980.1948.9917386.

McConnell, Susan. *Somatic Internal Family Systems Therapy: Awareness, Breath, Resonance, Movement, and Touch in Practice*. Berkeley: North Atlantic Books, 2020.

McGilchrist, Iain. *The Master and His Emissary: The Divided Brain and the Making of the Western World*. New Haven, CN: Yale University Press, 2019.

Nakken, Craig. *The Addictive Personality: Understanding the Addictive Process and Compulsive Behavior*. Center City, MN: Hazelden, 1996.

Netter, Frank H. *Atlas of Human Anatomy*. Philadelphia: Elsevier, 2011.

Newton, Michael. *Destiny of Souls: New Case Studies of Life Between Lives*. St. Paul, MN: Llewellyn Publications, 2000.

———. *Journey of Souls: Case Studies of Life Between Lives*. St. Paul, MN: Llewellyn Publications, 1994.

Ogden, Pat, and Janina Fisher. *Sensorimotor Psychotherapy: Interventions for Trauma and Attachment*. New York: W. W. Norton, 2015.

Ogden, Pat, Kekuni Minton, and Clare Pain. *Trauma and the Body: A Sensorimotor Approach to Psychotherapy*. New York: W. W. Norton, 2006.

Paulsen, Sandra. *Looking through the Eyes of Trauma and Dissociation: An Illustrated Guide for EMDR Therapists and Clients*. Bainbridge Island, WA: The Bainbridge Institute for Integrative Psychology, 2006.

Peirce, Penney. *Frequency: The Power of Personal Vibration*. New York: Atria Books, 2009.

Peate, Ian. *Anatomy and Physiology for Nursing and Healthcare Students at a Glance*. Hoboken, NJ: Wiley-Blackwell, 2022.

Pfender, April. *Reiki Healing for the Chakras: Techniques to Balance Your Mind, Body, and Spirit*. Oakland, CA: Rockridge Press, 2021.

Porges, Stephen W. "Emotion: An Evolutionary By-Product of the Neural Regulation of the Automatic Nervous System." *Annals of the New York Academy of Sciences* 807, no. 1 (December 2006): 62–77. https://doi.org/10.1111/j.1749-6632.1997.tb51913.x.

———. "Orienting in a Defensive World: Mammalian Modifications of Our Evolutionary Heritage. A Polyvagal Theory." *Psychophysiology* 32, no. 4 (July 1995): 301–318. https://doi.org/10.1111/j.1469-8986.1995.tb01213.x.

———. "The Polyvagal Perspective." *Biological Psychology* 74, no. 2 (February 2007): 116–143. https://doi.org/10.1016/j.biopsycho.2006.06.009.

————. *Polyvagal Safety: Attachment, Communication, Self-Regulation.* New York: W. W. Norton, 2021.

————. "The Polyvagal Theory: New Insights into Adaptive Reactions of the Automatic Nervous System." *Cleveland Clinic Journal of Medicine* 76, no. 4 (February 2009): 86–90. https://doi.org/10.3949/ccjm.76.s2.17.

————. *The Polyvagal Theory: Neurophysiological Foundations of Emotions, Attachment, Communication, and Self-Regulation.* New York: W. W. Norton, 2011.

————. "Vagal Pathways: Portals to Compassion." In *The Oxford Handbook of Compassion Science,* edited by Emma M. Seppälä, Emiliana Simon-Thomas, Stephanie L. Brown, Monica C. Worline, C. Daryl Cameron, and James R. Doty, 189–202. New York: Oxford University Press, 2017.

Porges, Stephen, and Deb Dana, eds. *Clinical Applications of the Polyvagal Theory: The Emergence of Polyvagal-Informed Therapies.* New York: W. W. Norton, 2018.

Quest, Penelope. *Reiki for Life: The Complete Guide to Reiki Practice for Levels 1, 2 & 3.* New York: Tarcher Perigee, 2016.

"Resources for Professionals and Students." Beck Institute. https://beckinstitute.org/cbt-resources/resources-for-professionals-and-students/.

Richo, David. *How to Be an Adult in Relationships: The Five Keys to Mindful Loving.* Boston: Shambhala, 2002.

Ruiz, Miguel. *The Four Agreements: A Practical Guide to Personal Freedom.* San Rafael, CA: Amber-Allen Publishing, 2018.

Sanossian, Nerses, and Sheryl Haut. "Chronic Diarrhea Associated with Vagal Nerve Stimulation." *Neurology* 58, no. 2 (January 2002): 330. https://doi.org/10.1212/WNL.58.2.330.

Saradananda, Swami. *Chakra Meditation: Discover Energy, Creativity, Focus, Love, Communication, Wisdom, and Spirit*. London: Watkins Publishing, 2011.

Schwartz, Arielle, and Barb Maiberger. *EMDR Therapy and Somatic Psychology: Interventions to Enhance Embodiment in Trauma Treatment*. New York: W. W. Norton, 2018.

Schwartz, Richard C. *Internal Family Systems Therapy*. New York: Guilford Press, 1995.

Schwartz, Richard C., and Martha Sweezy. *Internal Family Systems Therapy*. New York: Guilford Press, 2020.

Shannon, Nick, and Bruno Frischherz. *Metathinking: The Art and Practice of Transformational Thinking*. New York: Springer, 2020.

Shapiro, Francine. *Getting Past Your Past: Take Control of Your Life with Self-Help Techniques from EMDR Therapy*. Emmaus, PA: Rodale Books, 2012.

———. *Eye Movement Desensitization and Reprocessing (EMDR): Basic Principles, Protocols, and Procedures*. New York: Guilford Press, 2001.

Siegel, Daniel J. *The Developing Mind: How Relationships and the Brain Interact to Shape Who We Are*. New York: Guilford Press, 1999.

Sullivan, Marlysa B., Matt Erb, Laura Schmalzl, Steffany Moonaz, Jessica Noggle Taylor, and Stephen W. Porges. "Yoga Therapy and Polyvagal Theory: The Convergence of Traditional

Wisdom and Contemporary Neuroscience for Self-Regulation and Resilience." *Frontiers in Human Neuroscience* 12, no. 67 (February 2018). https://doi.org/10.3389/fnhum.2018.00067.

Suzuki, Shunryū. *Zen Mind, Beginner's Mind.* Edited by Trudy Dixon. Boston: Shambhala, 2006.

Tseng, Julie, and Jordan Poppenk. "Brain Meta-State Transitions Demarcate Thoughts Across Task Contexts Exposing the Mental Noise of Trait Neuroticism." *Nature Communications* 11 (July 2020). https://doi.org/10.1038/s41467-020-17255-9.

"Vagus Nerve." *Psychology Today.* Accessed 2022. https://www.psychologytoday.com/us/basics/vagus-nerve.

Wauters, Ambika. *Chakras and their Archetypes: Uniting Energy Awareness and Spiritual Growth.* Freedom, CA: Crossing Press, 1997.

Weiss, Brian L. *Directing Our Inner Light: Using Meditation to Heal the Body, Mind, and Spirit.* Carlsbad, CA: Hay House, 2020.

———. *Many Lives, Many Masters.* New York: Simon & Schuster, 1988.

Wilson, James L. *Adrenal Fatigue: The 21st Century Stress Syndrome.* Petaluma, CA: Smart Publications, 2001.

Zukav, Gary. *The Seat of the Soul.* New York: Simon & Schuster, 1989.